ENDING body burnout

FIND YOUR SPARK!

A functional medicine guide for "busy" women with energy, mood & gut issues

FILIPA BELLETTE, PHD
WITH CHRIS BELLETTE

Foreword by Lisa Corduff

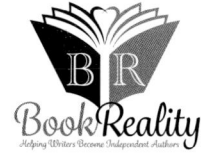

Copyright © Filipa Bellette, PhD 2023

Published: 2023 by The Book Reality Experience
Leschenault, Western Australia

ISBN: 9781923020108 - Paperback Edition
ISBN: 9781923020115 - eBook Edition

All rights reserved.

The right of Filipa Bellette, PhD to be identified as the author of this Work has been asserted by her in accordance with sections 77 and 78 of the Copyright, Designs and Patents Act 1988.

The information contained in this book is of a general nature and should not be regarded as legal advice or relied on for assistance in any particular circumstance or emergency situation. It is not intended as and should not be relied upon for medical advice. The publisher and author are not responsible for any specific health needs that may require medical supervision. If you have any underlying medical or mental health problems, or have any doubts about the advice contained in this book, you should contact a qualified medical, mental health or other appropriate professional.

The Publisher and author jointly or singularly, accept no responsibility or liability for any damage, loss or expense incurred as a result of the reliance on information contained in this guide.

Any third party views or recommendations included in this guide do not reflect the views of the Publisher, or indicate its commitment to a particular course of action.

No part of this publication may be reproduced, stored in a retrieval system, copied in any form or by any means, electronic, mechanical, photocopying, recording or otherwise transmitted without written permission from the publisher.

You must not circulate this book in any format.

Cover design and interior layout by Krysta Maria Micallef of www.xorxcreative.com from an original concept by the author.

Praise for Ending Body Burnout

'Ending Body Burnout translates complex science into digestible (pardon the pun) and practical information and strategies the reader can apply to better understand their health. Filly has distilled common health issues facing stressed and burned out women, into relatable case studies. This book is a must-read for any woman who's experienced burnout and is looking for science-backed solutions.'

Dr Kristy Goodwin | Speaker, Researcher, Author

'Burn out can be a bewildering place to be, and what we need in that place is expert information, a holistic approach and someone who has not only walked that path themselves, but has helped thousands of others do the same. Filipa, with this book, does exactly that.'

Lorraine Murphy | Best-Selling Author & Founder Lorraine Murphy

'There is so much to love about this book. And it's not just the fascinating exploration of applying Functional Medicine to our modern lives, or the set-by-step approach Filly takes. Nope, I think it's the humanness of this book that makes it a brilliant read. Science is great, but it's often inaccessible. Filly has a remarkable way of breaking things down and making them actionable. Ending Body Burnout. It's the book I'll be putting in the hands of everyone I know when she tells me she is confused about an aspect of her health.'

Lisa Corduff | Speaker & Founder Lisa Corduff

'This book is GOLD for any woman juggling all the things and stuck in the "B" word (busy!). After experiencing my own "body burnout" (gut issues, allergies, fatigue), I know just how much it can impact your ability to function in business and in life. Filipa's step-by-step process is what I wished I had, years ago'

Jeannie Savage | Founder Cloud 9 & Better in Business

'This book gives everyone an opportunity to take immediate steps towards being healthier and happier - regardless of where we are in life. Filipa's knowledge is shared in a relatable way through her real-life examples, and her genuine warmth really shines through the pages.

Having consulted with Filipa in the past, with great results for my health, I was excited to have many more "Wow!" moments as I read this book, and a feeling of being empowered to continue my journey. I wish I'd had access to the wisdom in this book, when I was a young, very burnt-out mum. I'm so glad to have the opportunity now as a woman in my fifties! Thanks Filly!'

Erica Mansfield | Tasmania, Australia

'Filipa Bellette, PhD has been an outstanding practitioner with a deep understanding of the field of functional medicine. I would encourage all who can to see her as a new client.'

Dr Daniel Kalish | Kalish Institute of Functional Medicine

Contents

Praise for Ending Body Burnout — 3
Contents — 5
Dedication — 7
Foreword — 9
Introduction — 13

Step One: The Body Systems — 21
   1. Neuroendocrine System — 29
   2. Gastrointestinal System — 45
   3. Detoxification System — 59

Step Two: Heal Thy Mind — 71
   4. Empowered Mind — 77
   5. Calm Mind — 97
   6. Organised Mind — 109

Step Three: Heal Thy Body — 121
   7. Restorative Nutrition — 125
   8. Restorative Sleep — 139
   9. Restorative Movement — 149

Step Four: Heal Thy Environment	159
10. Home Setup	163
11. Low Tox Home	171
12. Happy Home	185
Conclusion	197
References	203
Appendix	209
Acknowledgements	211
The Author	215

MEDICAL DISCLAIMER

This book is for informational purposes only. It is not a substitute for medical attention, treatment, examination, advice, treatment of existing conditions or diagnosis and is not intended to provide a clinical diagnosis nor take the place of proper medical advice from a fully qualified medical practitioner.

DEDICATION

This book is dedicated to my wonderful husband and business partner, Chris (who has contributed massively to this book), and our two spunky girls, Poppy and Elsie. And for every woman out there brave enough to deeply love herself!

Foreword

I was at an Awards night recently sitting with a highly accomplished friend. She's the mum of three, has a hugely successful career, looks on the outside to have it all together. But, like many women similar to her, she was struggling with confusing health issues.

She told me that she'd been working out daily at the gym and following 'healthy eating' plans but was exhausted all the time and gaining weight in a way that didn't make sense.

Her body was a mystery to her. She'd seen countless professionals and experimented with so many things and... nothing changed. It had been feeling really hopeless.

That night she shared she was feeling cautiously optimistic about the work she was doing with someone new.

The testing process, she told me, had been eye-opening in itself, with things being tested that she hadn't even considered were important. The lights were starting to go on. Could she really discover what was *actually* going on?

She mentioned the practitioners name was Filly.

Turns out it was the same Filly I'd been following on Instagram for a while. I loved the content I was seeing there.

What a refreshing take on health! What common sense! What a friendly face bringing burnt out women answers to questions that have eluded them for years. I felt excited for my friend. And curious too - I wondered if she'd get results.

It's a frustrating thing to be a woman who gets to mid-life, has achieved a lot, who has overcome hurdles, born children, figured things out - to crash face first into health issues that don't "make sense".

Or at least, they don't in the traditional medical model.

So we take it upon ourselves to research and experiment with all sorts of outside-the-box solutions but still, issues persist. Confusion reigns. It shouldn't be this way! It should not be this hard to feel good in a time when we have so much access to information.

And yet it is. Because no one is talking about body systems burning out.

As someone who has worked with thousands of women over the past decade helping them create positive change in their lives, the most common word I hear them use to describe how they feel is "overwhelmed". Life is too much.

In October 2022 I conducted "The Survey of Women: Stress, Sleep, Sex and More", and of the 1,430 respondents, only 1.8% felt fully rested. Which means 98.2% felt some level of tired.

It's crazy what we've normalised. And we are desperate for a roadmap out. Our bodies are begging us to pay attention.

Enter *Ending Body Burnout*. It's the book I'll be putting in the hands of everyone I know when she tells me she is confused about an aspect of her health.

This book is so needed right now. Burnout rates are skyrocketing.

Our generation knows so much. There's information everywhere. But it can feel like we are on a never-ending quest into the unknown. It's time-consuming, deflating and often very expensive!

There is so much to love about this book. And it's not just the fascinating exploration of applying Functional Medicine to our modern lives, or the set-by-step approach Filly takes.

Nope, I think it's the humanness of this book that makes it a brilliant read. Science is great, but it's often inaccessible. Filly has a remarkable way of breaking things down and making them actionable.

Not only that, following the three stories of Rose, Hazel and Isla readers will relate to their struggles and symptoms. And they can sigh with relief (like I did!) when the answers are presented clearly.

Functional Medicine is here to illuminate what's been hidden and there is no better person to serve burnt out women with this knowledge, than Filly.

She writes to educate, but it's her ability to educate AND empower that make this book something very special. Thank goodness for Filly bringing warmth and understanding.

Ending Body Burnout is not just the promise of actual results, but it contains the *proof* it can happen. For everyone.

Women deserve to feel better. Let this book be the start of a brand new revolution of wellness.

Lisa Corduff
www.lisacorduff.com

PS – That friend of mine who was cautiously optimistic she had found the right person to help her – turns out she got the answers and the results and will never look back.

Introduction

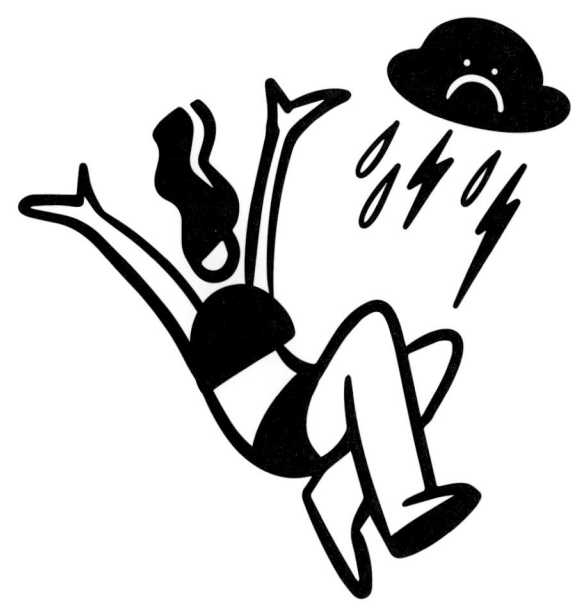

Hey there "busy" lady, juggling all the things! While busy-ness, overworking, addictive-doing & perfectionism might be the "norm" (and even a badge of honour) - it's NOT "normal". And it's a major contributor to health issues. And if you've got kiddies and a family to look after, that's adding even more into your already "overfull" schedule. First comes the physical stress of pregnancy, birth, breastfeeding, sleepless nights. Then, as the kids grow up, the mental load of juggling mothering, building a business or career, keeping your partner happy, housework, taxi-ing the kids, navigating teens, staying up late trying to tick-off your to-do's...It can be a recipe for disaster! All these stressors, if left unchecked, cause body burnout - meaning your body systems literally burnout, breakdown or become imbalanced.

If you're struggling with burnout symptoms like energy, mood and/or gut issues (especially if you're past the childbearing little baby years - or haven't even had kids), it is highly likely your insides aren't doing so well - and you'll want to listen up. So buckle in, and get ready for me to take you through, step-by-step, how you can rebuild your body and get your spark back - *without* giving up work, kids, and the things you love. Get ready for epic health well into your late 30's, 40's, 50's and beyond! Woot!

To get the most out of this book, start by taking our Ending Body Burnout Assessment - http://chrisandfilly.fm/scorecard. It will allow you to focus in on the areas of the book that are most beneficial to you when it comes to the extent of your body burnout, as well as the main root-cause contributors.

But before I dive into this book's concepts and suggestions, let me start by telling you my story.

My story

In 2012 I had my first baby. Poppy arrived after an intense five-year period completing my PhD, working in academia, and helping my hubby, Chris, build a business. Let's just say I was already "juggling all the things," and "burning the candle at both ends" - and this was *before* chucking kids into the mix. Poppy's birth was pretty traumatic. A long three-day labour, two hours of pushing, and forceps that ripped my vagina and part of my bowel a part. Oh, and my bladder stopped working. Like completely lost all sensation to pee, and I had to live with a catheter for the next three months. During this time I had lots of antibiotics, and was in-and-out of hospital with chronic constipation and urinary tract infections. Plus I was trying to look after a colicky baby that never stopped screaming (unless she was asleep). Over time I started developing more issues - fatigue, depression, anxiety, heartburn, low-immunity, skin issues, chronic sciatica pain, muscle weakness, chemical sensitivities.

When Poppy turned one, I knew my body would continue to fall a part, if I didn't do something. The GP's had been no help - all my blood test results were "fine." I was a new mum, apparently it was "normal" to feel burned-out. So I started taking my health into my own hands. I completely changed my diet. I ditched processed foods for whole foods. I was sprouting and fermenting and culturing and making everything from scratch. I even studied Nutritional Medicine and became a practitioner. I sought help from naturopaths, remedial therapists, energy healers. All these things helped to some extent, but still I didn't feel like I had reached the root of my issues. And when I had our second baby, Elsie, in 2015, all my symptoms flared up again - especially the anxiety. It reared its ugly head up with vengeance. I was angry, irritable, and on edge. I was the Dragon Mum. Screaming at my new born baby and toddler (and hubby!) all the time. I even started experiencing panic attacks. I'd completely lost the plot.

It scared me. I was deeply scaring myself. What type of mother had I become? If I didn't get a grip, I feared I'd end up psychologically damaging the kids, and getting a divorce. And I was a practising Clinical Nutritionist now - what type of practitioner was I, when I couldn't even sort myself out? How was I to keep a business running?

Then I found functional medicine - an integrative medicine approach that combines evidence-based functional lab testing with natural therapies to address body system imbalances and root-causes. It is the medicine of WHY - why are you sick in the first place? I was fascinated that I could test the health of my gut microbiome, my brain chemicals, hormones, mitochondria and detox pathways - body systems that go beyond what regular medical doctors test. And I was super excited that all these body systems could be healed using natural supplements, diet, lifestyle modifications, environmental changes and inner mind work. I did a mentorship with world-renowned USA-based functional medicine doctor, Dr Daniel Kalish, who first helped me to heal my body - and then to heal others. It was a game-changer!

There were ups and downs. Things that worked. And things that didn't. I also had a major health flare-up in 2020 when the COVID pandemic hit (more on that later). During this process of trial-and-error, I, along with my hubby Chris, who is also my business partner and our burnout recovery coach within our business (and contributing author to this book), created an award-winning method to end body burnout (for good!) in "busy" women and men. I'm the perfect person to be writing this because I was where you are now - and I now know how to get to the other side, without all the trial-and-error and wasting of time, money and sanity.

The other side

I see you, beauty, over there on the other side, where I once was. I really do. I see you juggling all the things. You're likely struggling with one - or perhaps all three - of these predominant health issues:

Fatigue issues

You're on the go all the time, hustling and grinding, trying to do all the things, keeping everyone happy, keeping everything afloat... and now you're exhausted, a Zombie, and your productivity at work is slipping. You'd so love to crash on the couch when you get home from work, but the dishes aren't done and the kids need to be fed. Sound familiar?

Mood issues

The exhaustion and overwhelm is all too much and you - snap! You're feeling anxious and irritable, struggling with hormonal mood swings, low libido, demotivated. You're feeling out of control, a Dragon Mum, a crabby wife, a short-tempered boss/colleague, and you keep wondering, "Is it all just in my head?"

Gut issues

When stress has been gnawing away at you, we often see gut issues erupt. Bloating, constipation, heartburn, diarrhoea, food sensitivities, or catching *all* the infections. For some people, other inflammatory symptoms will manifest too: headaches, period pain, acne, eczema, joint and muscle pain or autoimmunity. You start feeling broken, fragile, a shadow of what you used to be. You start losing joy in the life you live.

If these three main problems are left unchecked, things can quickly spiral. Physically you might get to the point where you struggle to function. You might struggle with the energy or mental capacity to work. You might have to quit your career or your business. You might struggle to payoff your mortgage. You might struggle to parent, or worry that Dragon Mum is going to screw up the kids - and/or your marriage. Body burnout can *cost you deeply.*

You may feel alone. But I promise you, you're not. In fact, data shows that working mother's are very susceptible to "burnout." While it is more commonly known that one out of five mothers develop post-natal depression in the first two years after childbirth, more recent data reveals that mothers juggling work and home-life face prolonged pressures and poor mental health, in particular anxiety, and physical burnout – regardless of a child's age or a woman's socio-economic background. In another study, 33% of mums say their career or work life has suffered after becoming a parent, and the same amount think their romantic relationship has deteriorated. The National Working Families Report showed that one quarter of working mothers are considering leaving their job in the next year due to stress caused by the conflict between work and caring responsibilities. Lisa Corduff, founder of The Change Room, also conducted a study in 2022 with 1430 women across the globe, and found that 98.2% don't feel fully rested, and that 56.8% rate their energy 5 or below out of 10. Burnout is real.

The solution

It may sound like "exhaustion" is the norm for "busy" women juggling all the things - but it's not normal, and it doesn't have to be this way. In fact, I wrote this book for *you* - and every other high-achieving woman out there. I wrote this book so that every human has the knowledge and the tools she needs to get her spark back, and end body burnout...for good! This is my life's purpose.

This book will help you discover the root-cause of your health issues. Modern medicine's quick-fix approach of "here, take this pill" does not work to address *why* you are feeling broken and burned-out in the first place. Popping an anti-depressant or sleeping pill might make you feel better, but it's not a long-term solution (and can actually make underlying issues worse). This book will also look at you as a WHOLE person. Unlike other health practitioners (medical and natural) who often treat "single pieces" of a person, our approach is to treat *all* of you, so you can heal at all levels - body, mind and environment - for complete resolution of body burnout and long-term health.

Throughout this book, I follow the stories of three women - Hazel, Isla and Rose - which give life to the many, sticky root-causes of body burnout. These women don't exist. They are a composite of stories from all the "busy" people we have worked with, struggling with body burnout after trying to juggle all the things. I've chosen to create composites, rather than tell individual client stories for two reasons: to protect the privacy of our clients, and to provide the scope to reflect the different conditions, circumstances and themes that high-achieving business owners and professional go-getters experience.

The real opportunity in this book, is that you will learn to love yourself, to care for your body and the way you think and feel about yourself, and to put yourself first. If you allow it, this book can be life-changing. You can have:

More energy
You'll get your spark back! You'll have a healthy, vibrant body, able to finally function, and feel alive again. Your body will be free of nasties. And you'll be in tune with what your body needs to stay well.

More productivity
You'll be more focused and purpose-driven. You'll have the energy required to build your business or career, and live your life the way you want to. You'll have more wisdom, balance and flow, able to achieve what you desire, without "doing more."

More connection
You'll be happier, and able to show up as a present and loving woman, mum, partner, boss, colleague, friend, because you're now loving yourself, fully, and backing yourself.

At the end of the day, honouring yourself first, is going to have a huge impact beyond just yourself. The work you do with this book is going to change not just yourself, but also your family, your business/career, the community, and the world. *And* you're going to have an impact on generations to come. If you don't get goosebumps thinking about that, I don't know what will!

The four-step method
Together with Chris, we have worked with more than 2000 burned-out women and men over the past combined two decades. We know a thing or two about overcoming and preventing burnout. Over the years, we've tested and fine-tuned what it takes to heal from body burnout, and end it...for good.

Ours is a four-step method.

Body systems
First, you need to find answers, a clear diagnosis, at the level of the body systems. This is Step One of this book. I'll show you how to identify which body systems have become imbalanced or burned-out, and causing your symptoms. Goodbye blank doctor stares after getting your blood test results back, showing all your results are "fine," when you don't "feel fine."

Heal thy mind
This is covered in Step Two of this book. If you ask why you are feeling burned-out in the first place, at the most honest, pared-back level, you will always discover the root-cause is due to how you think and feel about yourself. In Step Two, I delved into how your unconscious mind, your beliefs, thoughts and emotions are at the root-cause of your health issues, and what you need to do to address it.

Heal thy body
In Step Three of this book, I look into behaviour change in regards to how you eat, sleep and move. Unhealthy habits lead to body burnout. On the other hand, restorative healthy habits are powerful medicines. If healing the mind has been done correctly, you'll naturally want to behave in a loving way towards your body.

Heal thy environment
You do not live in a bubble. There are things in your environment, including people, that could be poisoning you or dragging you down. In the final section of this book, Step Four, I look at how you can set up and clean up your environment for optimal healing, health and happiness.

    I can't wait to dig deeper into all of this with you. Are you ready to get your spark back?
    Let's go!

STEP ONE
The Body Systems

STEP ONE
THE BODY SYSTEMS

Let's chat body systems. I could geek out on these guys all day. (Yep, I'm that nerd-of-a-mum who talks to her kids' friends during a playdate, all about gut bugs and brain chemicals!).

The first step to ending body burnout and getting your spark back, is to diagnose which body systems have "burned-out." This is what we call our Answers phase, and I can tell you it will save you a bucket-load of time, money and sanity. Why? Because many people try to treat their health issues with medication or supplements (either found on Dr Google or prescribed by a doctor or natural therapist, without any diagnostic reasoning), or by eating "healthy," joining a gym, or downloading a meditation app. While occasionally this helps, many people are left with unresolved burnout symptoms. You might get some improvement short-term, but your symptoms continue popping back. The reason for this is that very often there are bigger, underlying physiological imbalances that need repairing, and "eating well" or taking "magnesium" just won't do the trick - at least on their own.

In Step 1, I go over the three main body systems which can burnout, which then lead to symptoms, conditions, and eventually chronic diseases (let's get you well before you reach the point of diabetes or cancer!). The three body systems are: the Neuroendocrine System, the Gastrointestinal (GI) System, and the Detoxification System (as shown in figure 0.1).

I must acknowledge Dr Daniel Kalish of Kalish Institute of Functional Medicine, who mentored me in functional medicine for four years. This model is adapted from his Three Body Systems

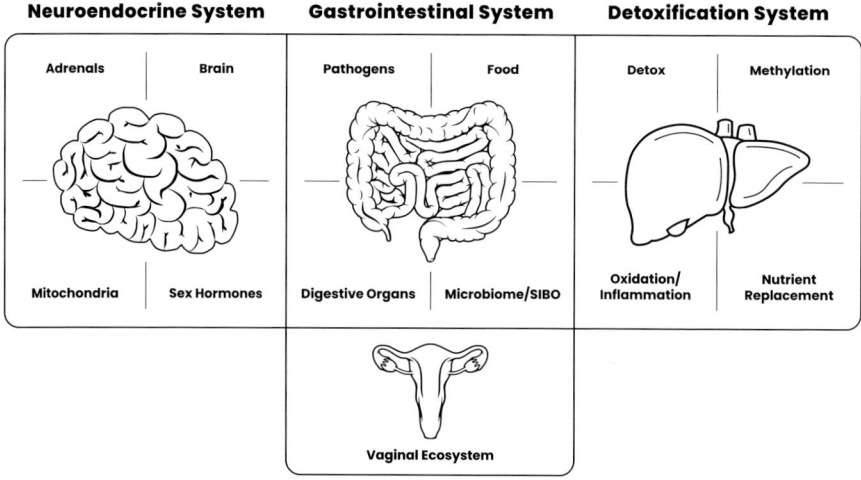

Figure 0.1: The Three Body Systems

Adapted from Dr Daniel Kalish, courtesy of the Kalish Institute

model - but with a Chris & Filly Functional Medicine twist. I literally had issues in all 17 areas (not even kidding!), so I don't just "textbook-know" how to test and treat them, I personally know.

Understanding which body systems have burned-out, as the first step, can help you feel better faster, as you know exactly what you need to do to restore proper function, and you get a clearer understanding of which root causes are at play. As you therapeutically reset your body systems, and you physically feel better, you will have the energy, motivation and mental clarity to do the stickier root cause work of addressing the mind, body and environment.

Before we dive into the body systems, let me first introduce you to Rose, Hazel and Isla.

Meet Rose, Hazel & Isla

Rose, Hazel and Isla
You're going to get to know these three ladies intimately throughout this book, and I'm sure you'll resonate with at least one of them (if not resonate with elements of all three!). To help you follow along with their ending body burnout journey, I've created a birds-eye view of all three that you can flick back to, in case you need a reminder of the conditions they are struggling with. You'll learn about the body system imbalances showing up in their lab tests, and the root-causes of their body burnout, throughout this book.

Handy tip you may want to dog-ear this page, to make it easier to flip back to!

Rose

Rose is a 38 year old mum of three, ages four, six and eight, and runs her own remedial therapy business from her rural home.

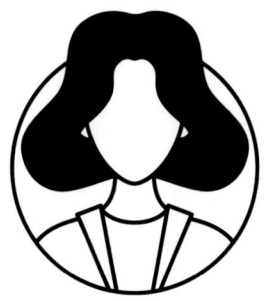

BODY BURNOUT SYMPTOMS

- Fatigue
- Brain fog
- Muscle weakness
- Difficulty falling to sleep
- Low mood
- Thrush and bacterial vaginosis
- Ringing in the ears
- Chronic "sniffles"

BODY SYSTEMS "BURNED-OUT" ON LAB TESTING

- Mitochondrial retraction
- Low dopamine
- Candida, bacterial vaginosis, parasites and low microbiome
- Methylation issues

KEY ROOT-CAUSES

- Hidden self-limiting beliefs around being "unlovable"
- People pleaser, motherhood martyrdom
- Sugar-addiction
- Burn-crash cycle with exercise
- Poor sleep hygiene
- Mould exposure

Hazel

Hazel is a 41 year old single mum, with two boys, 10 and 14 years, and works in a managerial corporate role.

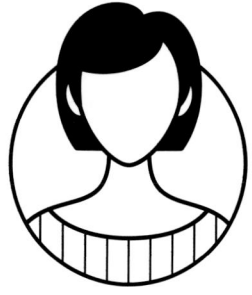

BODY BURNOUT SYMPTOMS

- Gut issues - bloating, alternating bowel movements
- Food sensitivities
- Heightened stress response
- Moody, irritable
- Low energy
- Itchy skin and eyes
- Random episodes of pins and needles

BODY SYSTEMS "BURNED-OUT" ON LAB TESTING

- Adrenal fatigue
- SIBO
- Leaky gut and digestive enzyme deficiency
- Inflammation of the gut, brain, and cellular level

KEY ROOT-CAUSES

- Hidden self-limiting beliefs around being "inadequate"
- Addictive-doing, over-working
- Proving & defending
- Eating on the run, poor food choices
- Sedentary

Isla

Isla is a 45 year old woman, owner of a busy, upmarket hair salon. She lives with her partner, and has no children.

BODY BURNOUT SYMPTOMS

- Anxiety
- Struggles to breath, chest pain
- Heartburn
- Broken sleep, nightmares
- Weight gain
- Heavy, painful period
- Hot flushes
- History of infertility

BODY SYSTEMS "BURNED-OUT" ON LAB TESTING

- Low serotonin
- Estrogen dominance
- H.pylori and high beta-glucoronidase
- Bile production issues
- Hiatal hernia
- Detox pathways depleted

KEY ROOT-CAUSES

- Hidden self-limiting beliefs on feeling "unworthy"
- Past trauma
- Easily distracted, running away
- Yoyo dieting, restrictive eating, binge eating
- Over-exercising
- High toxin exposure

CHAPTER 1
Neuroendocrine System

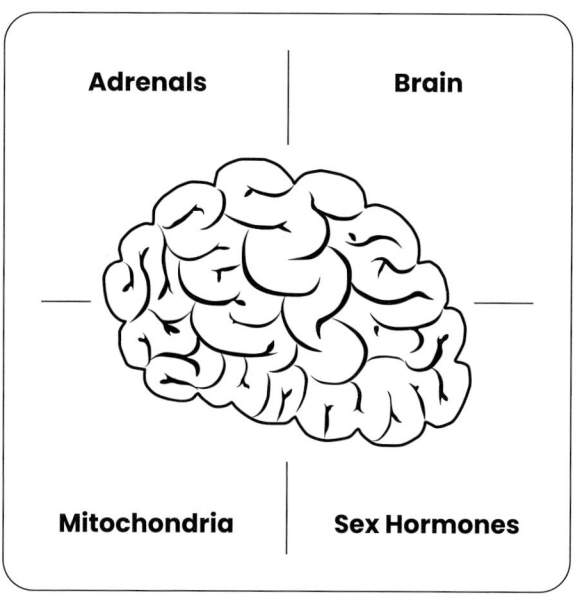

Introduction

In this chapter, you'll learn all about the neuroendocrine system, and the four main areas that make up this system - the adrenals, the brain, the mitochondria and the sex hormones.

Essentially, this system controls how you think, feel and act. It's also very important for controlling and regulating the major functions and processes of the body, including energy production and reproduction. If you're a "busy" woman with a never-ending to-do-list, your neuroendocrine system is likely getting a thrashing. You've probably heard the saying: "I'm living on adrenaline" or "my adrenals are fried." These terms are often thrown about by high-achievers juggling all the things. And they are right - you are likely burning through your adrenaline (brain chemical) and frying your adrenals (depleting your stress hormones).

In this chapter, you'll get a clear understanding of what the areas in the neuroendocrine system actually are, why they're important, how they burnout, and how to know if your neuroendocrine system needs some TLC.

Adrenals - Hazel's were fried

Hazel was, let's just say, burning the candle at both ends.

"I'm sick of feeling like crap," she said bluntly, sitting in front of me, staring me down. Hazel wasn't the type of woman you'd want to double-cross. And while her hard-core personality got her up the corporate ladder, it most likely burned-out her adrenals too.

"My gut's a mess. I can't eat anything. I'm exhausted. And stress is really getting the better of me," she said, tapping her foot.

Hmm, foot tapping. Lot's of pent-up, anxious energy there.

"How's stress showing up for you, Hazel?" I asked.

"My kids! Ergh, my kids are triggering me every second. Which I just hate, because I hardly see them. You know, work, it's so flat out. Even when I'm at home, I'm trying to complete a million things. But. Ergh! I'm just so snappy at my boys all the time. And even at work, little things I used to be able to tolerate, are just driving me insane. And trying to do more than one project at a time. I just can't do it anymore. And I'm forgetting things," Hazel said, shoulders slumped. "I'm not usually like that. I usually have all my stuff together."

"Can I tell you about the adrenal glands?" I asked.

"Sure, if you think it's going to help."

I sure do Hazel. I sure do.

The adrenals sit on top of your kidneys, and one of their major roles is to regulate your stress hormones: cortisol and dehydroepiandrosterone (big word, I know. Let's shorten it to DHEA). When you're under stress, the brain tells the adrenal glands to secrete cortisol, which causes your body to respond to stress.

When there is enough cortisol flooded in the blood, the brain then sends a signal to the adrenals to secrete DHEA, which in effect brings cortisol levels (and you!) back down to a relaxed state.

Now let's imagine your stress-load is like a bucket that you can fill up and empty. There are many types of stressors that can fill your bucket up. Most people only think of emotional stressors (Hazel had a lot of these!), but other things will put stress on your adrenal glands, like pathogens in the gut, environmental toxins, temperature discomfort, exercise, multi-tasking, over-doing, lack of sleep, sugar, processed foods, electromagnetic fields (EMF's - also known as "dirty electricity"), unexpected change, and even exciting things like planning for a wedding or a holiday.

To empty the bucket, you need to reduce stressors and add in recovery activities - get lots of sleep, eat nutritious foods, spend time in nature, do yoga, meditate, think healthy thoughts about yourself, laugh, play, stop and just lie in the sun, detox, and reduce inflammation in the gut. If the stressors are filling up the bucket too fast, in comparison to emptying your bucket, you will start producing an overload of cortisol.

Over time, when there is *too much* cortisol being secreted, DHEA levels will start depleting, as it can no longer keep up with its crazy, hyperactive counterpart.

What happens then, when DHEA is no longer being secreted efficiently?

There is no hormone to balance cortisol and bring you back down to a state of calm.

It is absolutely *crazy* how common this hormonal dysfunction is happening. I'd say 80-90% of our clients tested for adrenal fatigue, come back as positive.

Hazel's incessant foot tapping slowed down, and she started to nod. "Ok, so my crazy, busy life is causing my adrenals to burnout?"

"Yes!" I said. "Well that's my hunch. We'll have to test to confirm."

Hazel sat back, crossing her arms. Her eyes narrowed. "So why hasn't my GP tested my adrenals. He ran a gazillion tests. He never mentioned anything about the adrenals?"

Ahh, the good old medical system, letting people like Hazel slip through the cracks again. I cleared up Hazel's concerns (dare I say suspicions about testing the adrenals), by explaining to her that many GP's (unless they are a medical doctor specialising in functional medicine) disregard the adrenals as contributing to body burnout symptoms. They will likely tell you that "adrenal fatigue" is not real, and will only say adrenals are an issue if you have a serious adrenal disease, like Cushing's Syndrome or Addison's Disease (where the body either produces drastically too much or too little of your stress hormones). These diseases are pretty rare, and are diagnosed by an endocrinologist. Because the term "adrenal fatigue" is a bit elusive, many conventional medical doctors do not consider stress hormone imbalance a "thing." James Wilson, in his book *Adrenal Fatigue*, rightly states that low adrenal function has become "invisible" to modern medicine. While your adrenals can't literally become "fatigued," the hormones the adrenals produce can definitely become dysfunctional.

The thing is, the adrenals play a huge role in symptom and disease onset, and are often the first part of the body that breaks down, which then leads to a cascade of other symptoms and conditions. Many - and I mean *many!* - juggling high-achievers (and not just women, men as well) are walking around with taxed adrenals. I was one of them - and so was my husband and business partner Chris! And while many of these people don't have a full-blown adrenal disease like Cushing's Syndrome or Addisons's Disease, their imbalanced stress hormone production are absolutely manifesting as energy, mood, gut and other inflammatory issues.

The adrenal glands are responsible for not just dealing with stress, however, but also for resiliency, energy, and endurance. When your adrenal stress hormones burnout, your entire body feels it and suffers from exhaustion. Common symptoms associated with adrenal fatigue are abnormal stress response, anxiety, depression, low energy, brain fog, female hormones issues (i.e. PMS, irregular cycle, infertility, peri/menopausal symptoms), insomnia, low-immunity, lower back pain, and gut issues.

Hazel nodded her head as I showed her a diagram of symptoms associated with adrenal fatigue. "I have almost all of those symptoms!" she cried. "How do we test these annoying hormones?"

I laughed. "Your adrenal glands aren't annoying, Hazel. They might just *feel* annoying right now. But once we get them fixed up, you'll have a new-found love and respect for these important glands."

I pulled out my basket of functional lab tests. "My big philosophy when it comes to ending body burnout is to 'test not guess,'" I said.

"You know I'm not here to stuff around!"

When it comes to testing for adrenal fatigue, we use an AdrenoCortex Stress Profile saliva test from Nutripath (check out Appendix for more info). All you have to do is fill up a 5ml tube with saliva (I know, it's quite a lot of saliva) four times in a day. Testing, rather than guessing, will save you so much time and money. Prior to specialising in functional medicine, I would place clients on an adrenal protocol purely based on their symptoms, case history and my educated guesswork. For some people, the underlying cause of their symptoms actually wasn't due to adrenal fatigue at all. The treatment was all wrong, and of course, they got little benefit.

Hazel did her saliva sample, and sure enough, a week or two later, her test results showed adrenal fatigue.

"How do we fix it?" Hazel asked, her eyes sparking with hope for the first time.

Hold on Hazel - and dear reader - we'll get to that soon! But first, let's look at the brain.

Brain - Rose's was depleted

When I first met Rose, I could see the exhaustion in her whole body. Her skin was dull. Her eyes clouded. Her words were slow and disjointed. Even the way she walked and sat was "tired." Rose was struggling with fatigue, big time, as well as brain-fog, low mood, sleep issues, thrush, and muscle weakness.

"I have no get-up-and-go. I'm so exhausted all the time. And I just can't seem to do the things I know I should be doing to be healthy." Rose was almost in tears.

"Like what?" I asked.

"Like not eating a block of chocolate at night, for a start! I just feel so flat. And not just physically. It feels like a real mental flatness. I know what I should be doing, but I have no motivation."

This was a hard thing for Rose, working as a massage therapist. There she was, talking to her clients all day about living in a way to reduce inflammation, yet she couldn't stop binging out on sugar.

"I saw the GP a few months back. It was a waste of time. He said all my bloods looked 'fine' and that it's normal for a mum to feel like this, especially with three young kids."

Um, no Mama! It is not normal! Reader, if you ever get this flip-off response, don't accept it. It is not normal to feel crappy after having kids. It may be the "norm," yes, but it's not normal.

"I've been taking a bunch of supplements from a Naturopath I saw awhile ago. She said they were for stress - adrenals maybe? But to tell you the truth, I don't feel any better."

"Did you get tested for adrenal fatigue?" I asked.

"No, I think it was just based on my symptoms...maybe?"

"Well," I said, "it's probably because the adrenals aren't the issue. Can I talk to you about the brain?"

Like the adrenals, the brain gets a big hit in busy women, juggling all the things. In our practice, we test and treat four main important neurotransmitters: adrenaline, noradrenaline, dopamine and serotonin. The first three neurotransmitters are your "get-up-and-go" brain chemicals. They are super important for energy and motivation. In this way, they function a bit like your stress hormone cortisol. Dopamine is also your "feel good" neurotransmitter, and plays a role in feeling creativity, joy and self-confidence. Serotonin is important for good sleep and a balanced mood. When any of these neurotransmitters deplete, it can lead to anxiety, depression, fatigue, brain fog, insomnia, lack of motivation, restless legs, shakiness, and even addictive type behaviour, like food addictions/disorders, alcoholism, smoking, repetitive thought or behavioural patterns, and even full-blown OCD.

I told Rose a story, to show her how brain chemical depletion plays out in real life.

When I tested my brain, it showed low dopamine levels. And I was feeling it. I struggled to feel joy and excitement. An example: when I finished my PhD, I should've been over the moon, booking a celebratory holiday to Bali. But instead I felt flat, indifferent, and thought, *what's next?* I was also showing addictive tendencies. When my anxiety was at it's all time high, I started displaying irrational and repetitive thoughts about Chris. I needed to monitor everything he was doing, who he was seeing, who he was talking too, and even checking his emails and messages. When I started healing my depleted brain, within a few weeks I had no - absolutely no - desire to do this anymore. It was like I woke up and thought: *well that was a waste of time, Filly!*

"My addictive tendency is sugar!" Rose blurted.

Just as the adrenals burnout due to too much stress, so do the neurotransmitters. Over-doing, working too much, juggling too many things, not sleeping enough, and emotional stress and trauma can all cause your brain chemicals to burnout. Indulging in addictive habits - even over-exercising - can also highjack your brain chemicals.

Rose nodded her head. "I have had a lot of stress in the past. And the kids have really disrupted my sleep patterns. And maybe I used to exercise too much?"

Just wait Rose, there are more root causes...

Concussions or a bad knock to the head can damage your brain chemicals, so can environmental toxins. And sometimes the cause of brain chemical depletion is due to poor diet or gut health. You see, amino acids (protein from food), like tyrosine and tryptophan, support your neurotransmitters. If you are on a very low-protein diet, or not eating all your essential amino acids, you may be damaging your brain. Most people (even vegans) eat enough protein, however. And it's more likely that you're not actually breaking down and absorbing protein in your gut. Genetic issues can also underlie brain issues.

"Gee, maybe my brain *is* messed up!" Rose said, with a little smile. The first proper smile I'd seen. Clarity and hope always makes even the most fatigued person perk up.

"To really know, we'll have to test your brain," I said, pulling out an organic acids urine test kit (check out Appendix for more info on Nutripath testing).

"What? You can test my brain with wee!"

"I'm excited you're excited, Rose. I think it's pretty darn cool you can see the health of your neurotransmitters with a splash of wee."

"I can't believe no one's ever asked to test my brain? It makes so much sense, considering how I'm feeling. Instead I was treated for adrenal fatigue - and that didn't do much."

Unfortunately, the brain is rarely investigated. Medical doctors don't test this important part of the body. If you're struggling with anxiety or depression or even fatigue, you'll usually just get prescribed an anti-depressant, without any investigative testing. Even neurologists and psychiatrist don't test your dopamine or adrenaline or serotonin levels (why this isn't a routine test, I don't know!). Many natural therapists don't look at this area either. Many clients have come to us after seeing a different nutritionist or naturopath or even a functional medicine practitioner, and the brain has never been mentioned. For many of these clients, doing brain work made *all* the difference.

When Rose got back her urine test and it revealed low dopamine, she started to cry. "I'm so sorry," she said. "I was starting to feel like there was no hope for me. Thank you for giving me hope."

Thank you Rose for never quitting. But just wait, Rose. There's more. We need to look at your mitochondria next.

Mitochondria - Rose's story continues

Rose didn't just have brain issues. She also had burned-out mitochondria, which was tested using the same organic acids test.

Mito-say-whaaaat?! Let me tell you all about these guys.

The mitochondria are tiny organelles that live in your muscle tissue, and their role is to convert food - specially fats, proteins and carbs - into Adenosine 5-triphosphate (another big word again, let's call it ATP) energy. Hello energy again! ATP is the principle molecule for storing and transferring energy in cells. It is often referred to as the energy currency of the cell and can be compared to storing money in a bank. If your mitochondria aren't doing so well, you could be left feeling very fatigued. Other symptoms I commonly see with mitochondrial issues are post-exercise fatigue (you feel worse and more exhausted after physical exercise, as opposed to brighter), weight gain (if you're not converting food into energy effectively, the food gets stored in your fat tissues), and a general feeling of weakness or achiness.

"Is that why I feel *even more* exhausted after exercise?" Rose asked, hands outstretched.

"Yes, it definitely could be! Your low energy and motivation could be coming from low dopamine, but when you're getting post-exercise fatigue as well, I start putting a little question mark over the mitochondria."

Not being able to exercise like she used to, was a real sticking point for Rose. Before having kids, Rose was super fit and active. She ran 10km a few times a week, went to the gym, did yoga, and was even on a basketball team. But after kids, when her energy levels crashed, doing a thirty minute walk exhausted her - and it wasn't improving, even as the kids grew up.

"Is that why I feel wiped out after massaging clients all day, too?"

"Yes, most likely. Any physical movement can make you feel worse, if your mitochondria aren't in good health."

"So what caused this - having babies?" Rose laughed.

"Well, yes, that would've put a strain on your body. But there are most likely other things at play."

Having kids can put a physical stress on your body and cause you to burn through nutrients. Nutrient deficiency is one major way the mitochondria can become imbalanced. You need a bunch of important nutrients - like carnitine, vitamin B's, magnesium, CoQ10 - that are needed to convert fats, proteins and carbs into ATP energy. If any of these nutrients become deficient you can't convert foods into energy very effectively. And yes, using lab testing we can see exactly which nutrients are deficient. Common causes for this are genetic issues, poor diet or gut issues (as in, you're not eating enough of the important mitochondria micronutrients, or you're not digesting them very well), or there is a lot of inflammation in your body and you're burning up micronutrients trying to protect yourself from further damage.

The other major way the mitochondria becomes imbalanced is when the actual organelles are damaged. In a lab test, we can actually see how damaged the mitochondria are - some people are only showing 25-50% mitochondrial function. If you only have 25-50% of your mitochondria functioning, of course there are going to be energy issues. It's like only driving a four cylinder car, with only one or two cylinders operating. Things that cause the mitochondria to become damaged are over-exercising, environmental toxins, mould and pathogens, especially viral pathogens like Epstein Barr virus (glandular fever) and COVID-19.

When I mentioned glandular fever, Rose's eyes widened. "I had glandular fever after having my first baby and I've never felt the same since! And mould - holy crap! We moved into our farm house about the same time. I'm sure there's hidden mould in the old house."

Connecting the dots - I love it.

Sex hormones - Isla's were all over the place

Isla desperately wanted answers. I could see it in her eyes, even via our online video consult. She was struggling with many body burnout symptoms, but her biggest complaint were her hormonal issues. Ever since she was a teen, she suffered with heavy, painful periods. She'd been prescribed all sorts of contraceptives to try to address the periods, but they all made her feel worse - "like a crazy woman" - Isla had said. And she'd never been able to fall pregnant, even after rounds of IVF.

"My only option was to live with the heavy, painful periods - with lots of Ibuprofen, mind you! - but now I'm starting to get other hormonal issues. Hot flushes. And also weight," she said, grabbing her belly. "I've always been trim around the middle, but lately the weight seems to be stacking on."

"Sounds like you might be peri-menopausal," I suggested.

"Yes! That's what all my girlfriends have said."

Figure 1.1: Female Hormone Menstrual Cycle

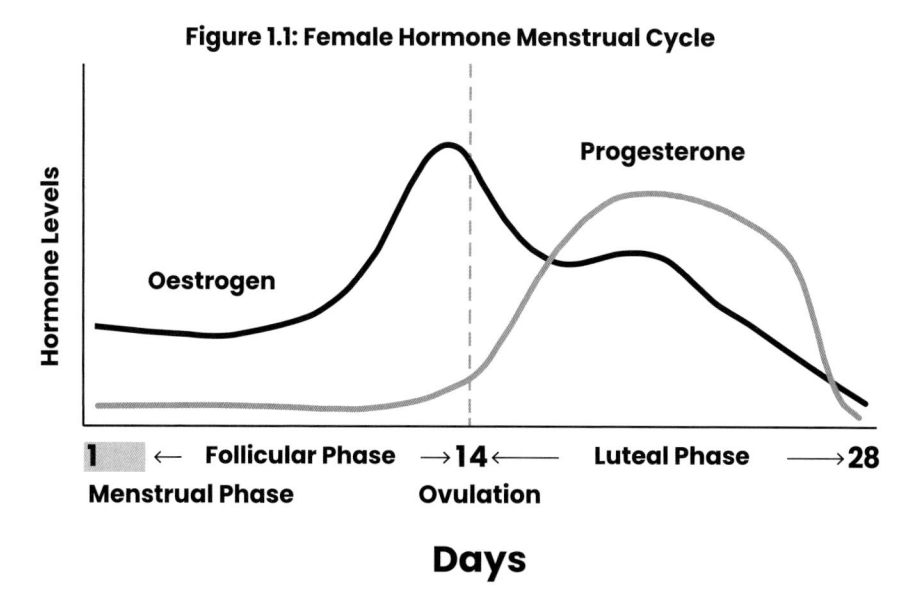

Fig 1.1 Female hormone menstrual cycle

"The thing is, Isla, peri/menopausal symptoms, as well as period and PMS issues in general, might be the 'norm', but they aren't normal. It's a strong sign that your hormones are out of whack. And the fact you struggled with infertility, is more evidence of that."

To dive into what this actually looks like, I have to first show you what balanced hormones look like. By balanced, I'm talking about the ratio of your oestrogen and progesterone hormones, as well as testosterone (yes, ladies need testosterone, too, to function optimally). Let's start looking at what your oestrogen and progesterone levels should be doing over a healthy 28 day menstrual cycle (as shown in figure 1.1).

Isn't that a dance of hormonal beauty? In the follicular phase, hormone production is pretty low, initially. Then oestrogen starts to rise, and peaks at day 14, which causes ovulation and the release of an ova, or egg. Ta da! Hello little egg!

If there is no sperm present (or if Mr Sperm missed the boat) to fertilise the egg, oestrogen will start to drop in the second half of the cycle, and progesterone will rise. As the cycle nears the end of the 28 days, both progesterone and oestrogen drop, which then gives way to the beautiful gush of blood, which is your period (beautiful, that is, only if these hormones are dancing and fluctuating as they should be).

"Sounds like my hormones aren't going to win 'Dancing with the Stars' anytime soon," Isla joked.

I agree, Isla. There has to be something out-of-sync, in order to cause painful, heavy periods and infertility. Any disruption with the hormones for a menstruating woman can also lead to PMS symptoms, irregular cycle, mood swings, headaches, migraines, fatigue, sugar cravings, pimples, diarrhoea or constipation, sore breasts, facial hair, and low sex-drive.

If the hormones are already out-of-balance, things can go even more pear-shaped when a woman enters perimenopause, as the hormones start to drop unevenly. Lara Briden, hormone expert, calls perimenopause the "second puberty", and can last as long as two to ten years leading up to a woman's last period (menopause), and start as early as the late 30's. Just as it's "not normal" to have painful periods and PMS, neither is it "normal" to have perimenopausal symptoms: hot flushes, mood imbalances, night sweats, insomnia, or weight gain (beyond an extra 5kg).

So how do the female hormones go pear-shaped in the first place?

Sex hormones are delicate petals, and there are many things that can tip them over the edge. Stress is a big one. The sex hormones are closely linked to your stress hormones, cortisol and DHEA (remember the adrenal glands from earlier in this chapter? Yep, those guys). DHEA converts into oestrogen and testosterone, and cortisol, when secreting in high amounts due to stress, directly suppresses progesterone production. It's very common to see an imbalance in both the stress and sex hormones. And likewise, all the myriad of stressors that cause adrenal imbalances, can also affect the sex hormones - an inflammatory diet, caffeine, alcohol, sugar, emotional stress, pregnancy, birth, sleepless nights, trauma, environmental toxins, cleaning and skincare products, over-working/doing, mould, gut inflammation, medications and contraceptives.

"But didn't my adrenal test come back fine?" Isla said, her eyes squinted in confusion.

Yep, crazily enough, Isla's adrenals were functioning text-book perfect. For Isla, there were other "stressors" at bay.

Enter: detox isses. Dum, dum, dummmmm.

Poor detoxification is also a very common cause of hormone imbalance, especially when it comes to having *too much* oestrogen. One of the liver's many jobs is to metabolise and excrete excess hormones, especially oestrogen. If the liver is under stress, sluggish, or burning out, it's always going to work on priority number one: clearing dangerous toxins from your body. That means oestrogen clearance will take the back seat. Your body knows clear-well that you can survive ok with imbalanced hormones, but if you're riddled with poisons, well, you may as well start digging an early grave.

Gut issues can also cause hormonal imbalances. Any inflammation in the gut, will cause stress to your adrenals, which can then drag progesterone down. Likewise, there are very specific bacteria in the gut - ß-glucuronidase - which bind onto oestrogen. Rather than eliminating excess hormones via the bowels, the bacteria recirculate oestrogen back into your system, increasing the total amount of oestrogen in the body.

"Are you serious? My hormones could be out-of-whack because of some nasty bacteria?!" Isla said, eyes wide.

Yes Isla, but that's not the only thing. Detox issues for her, were also a major cause. I'll talk more about this later.

We tested Isla's sex hormones using a 28 day female hormone saliva test from Nutripath (check out Appendix for more info). Basically she filled a test tube up with saliva every two or three days, so that we could measure the rhythm of her progesterone and oestrogen over the course of a whole cycle, plus test her testosterone levels.

Isla had said to me, when I suggested doing this test: "but my GP already ran some bloods and she said all my hormone markers looked fine."

I cringed. I get this remark all the time. The issue with only taking one blood sample to look at female hormones is that you miss critical information about what's happening over the course of the whole cycle. While Isla's one blood sample looked "fine" (it must of caught her hormones on an ok day), when we got her full 28 day female hormone results back, we could see the full picture of her very fluctuating (in an abnormal way) hormones. Sure enough, she was producing very little progesterone in the second half of her cycle, and her oestrogen levels were zipping up and down, up and down, over the cycle, with the ratio of oestrogen being much higher than progesterone.

"That, Isla, is what we call oestrogen dominance, and it can for sure cause major sex hormone issues."

Isla sat back on her seat and let out a big breath. A breath that had been stuck inside of her for decades. Answers. She was finally getting some answers.

Throughout this chapter, you have seen through the experiences of our busy women, Hazel, Rose and Isla, how imbalances in the neuroendocrine system can lead to body burnout symptoms, and how you can test these areas to confirm imbalances. You've also discovered some root causes, that cause the neuroendocrine system to burnout in the first place. We'll dive deeper into these, later in the book.

Next up, is one of my favs: the gastrointestinal system. (Actually, they're all my favs!).

SUMMARY
NEUROENDOCRINE SYSTEM

In this chapter, you have learned about the four body systems that make up the neuroendocrine system:

The Adrenals
Your stress hormones cortisol and DHEA

The Brain
Your neurotransmitters adrenaline, noradrenaline, dopamine and serotonin

The Mitochondria
The organelles in your muscle tissue that convert food into energy

The Sex Hormones
Progesterone, oestrogen and testosterone

CHAPTER 2
Gastrointestinal System

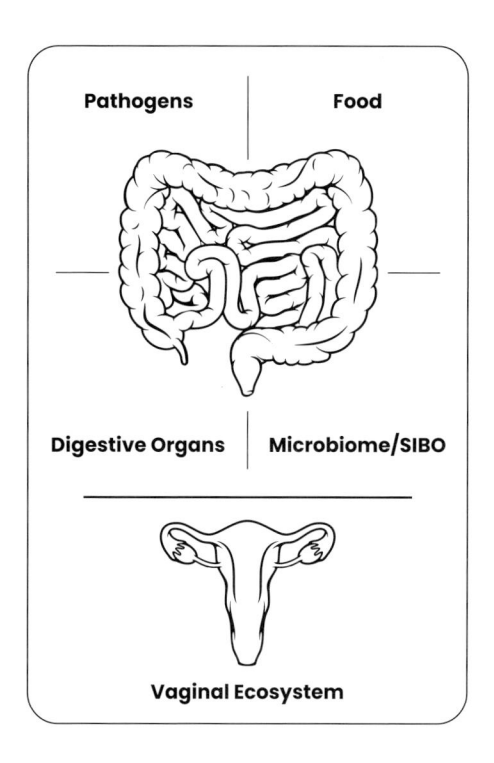

Diagram showing four quadrants labeled Pathogens, Food, Digestive Organs, Microbiome/SIBO around an illustration of the intestines, with a Vaginal Ecosystem illustration below.

Introduction

In this chapter, you'll learn all about the gastrointestinal (GI) system, and the four main areas that make up this system - pathogens, digestive organs, microbiome/SIBO and the vaginal ecosystem (ok, not part of the gut, technically, but there is a strong link between the gut bugs and the vaginal bugs). You'll notice "food" is also part of the GI system, but I'm going to chat about food later, in Chapter 7.

Dr Michael Gershon, father of neurogastroenterology, coined the GI system "the second brain." The gut has a strong link with the neuroendocrine system; it is constantly sending signals through the nervous system up to the brain (and vice versa). Have you ever felt emotionally stressed, and your gut has started squirming? Yep, that's the gut-brain connection right there. So imagine if you're running around with your never-ending to-do list and screaming kids, overwhelmed and stressed-out, what exactly is happening down there in the gut? It's likely breaking down.

The GI system is also the central place where you breakdown and absorb foods. If anything goes wrong with the gut, you'll struggle to absorb the nutrients that other body systems need to function. Which leads to further body system burnout, and yep, more exhaustion, mood imbalances and inflammatory symptoms.

In this chapter, you'll get a clear understanding of what the areas in the GI system actually are, why they're important, how they burnout, and how to know if your GI system needs some love.

Get ready for lots of talk about poo and pathogens, and fungi growing in your bum (or vagina!).

Pathogens - welcome back, Rose

Squirmy worms. Pesky parasites. Cunning candida. Bothersome bacteria. They might be tiny in size, but holy moly these gut pathogens can cause tyranny - and not just in the gut, but in your whole body.

No one likes seeing worms or parasites show up on their lab tests. Rose cringed when she saw the little fella, blastocystis hominis, show up on her labs. "I swear I wash my hands!"

"It's ok, Rose, I believe you," I laughed. "It's actually surprisingly common for people to have parasites. They're often picked up from drinking tank water, river water, or even from unwashed fruit or veggies. And yep, you could also get it from ingesting poo - other peoples, or animals."

Rose shuddered. "I will be more diligent scrubbing the chook eggs before I bring them into the kitchen!"

When it comes to parasites and worms, there are some pretty nasty ones that you definitely don't want to see in a lab test. Giardia is a good example. It's extremely inflammatory, and can feel like it's ripping your gut raw (that's not an exaggeration, by the way). Other parasites and worms can be more benign, and if your gut is reasonably balanced and healthy, you could live in blissful harmony together. Research also shows they can also help assist the immune system. But, if your immune system is suppressed, and your microflora is generally dysbiotic (i.e. not enough good bugs and too many bad bugs), then these more benign worms and parasites can overgrow and cause significant issues. A few reasons for this: parasites and worms can borrow into the intestinal lining, and create "holes" in the gut lining - *and* other organs (eek!). Some also spit out toxic metabolites that inflame the gut. And lastly, parasites and worms can cause nutritional deficiencies because, well, they can munch up all the food you're eating, before you can actually absorb the nutrients.

"So even if I'm eating the best, healthiest diet, my body might not be getting any of the nutrients?" Rose asked.

"Exactly!"

"No wonder I feel so depleted all the time," Rose said, slumping back in her chair.

But Rose didn't just have a parasite infection, she also had a yeast infection. Or more specifically: candida. Parasites and candida are not a good combo. Hidden parasites often feed chronic candida issues that don't seem to clear up.

Candida is part of the normal flora, but it can quickly overgrow if given the right opportunity, like post-antibiotics, or while on medications like the contraceptive pill, or scoffing too much gluten, alcohol or sugar (ah hem - possibly a root cause right there, dear Rose!). Like parasites, candida and other fungi infections spit out toxic metabolites, specifically acetaldehyde, which has alcoholic properties. "Alcohol" floating around in your system 24/7 is never going to be a good thing. You basically become an alcoholic (without knowing it!), living constantly with a chronic hangover.

"Yes! I've never thought about it like that, but you've hit the nail on the head," Rose cried. "My exhaustion, lethargy, brain fog, low mood - it's like I'm waking up every morning with a bad hangover after a big night on the town!"

These are common symptoms that arise due to pathogen infections. Many other clients we have worked with also experience gut related symptoms, like diarrhoea, bloating, abdominal pain, heartburn, constipation, blood and mucous in the stool. Anxiety, depression, achiness, allergies, low-immunity, hormonal imbalances and skin issues are also very common.

In lab tests, we can also pick up nasty bacterial and viral pathogens, like h.pylori, c. difficile toxin A & B and e.coli. I personally struggled with a h.pylori infection, which showed up in the past as chronic heartburn. When I did my own stool test, I literally cried happy tears to find h.pylori, as I'd been struggling with treatment-resistant heartburn for the past 15 years. Clearing up the h.pylori took the fire from my chest - it also dramatically improved my anxiety and low-immunity issues (at least initially - more on my heartburn flare-up soon!).

Stool test - yep, that's how these pathogenic microbes are found. In our practice, we mostly use a PCR complete microbiome mapping stool test from Nutripath (check out Appendix for more info). PCR technology uses chemicals to look at the DNA of species in the stool. Even if microbes die off in the mail from your house to the pathology labs, the DNA of these little critters will still be found. You might be thinking - but doesn't my GP test for pathogens? Yes, they do test the six or so most common parasites and bacterial pathogens, but that's about it. GP's rarely test for worms or candida overgrowth in the gut. Plus the standard medical stool test misses pathogens that might not be considered an "issue" in modern medicine, but in actual fact can cause some serious functional health issues.

Digestive organs - hello again, Isla

Isla's digestive organs weren't doing so well. We could see clearly on her labs.

Digestive organs are the organs in the gut that help breakdown and absorb food, and keep your immune system and overall body functioning well. These include: the stomach, the pancreas, the gall bladder and the gut lining.

Isla, if you remember from the previous chapter, was struggling with female hormone issues. On her labs, it showed she was struggling to breakdown fats from her food, which is common to see when the gallbladder isn't squirting sufficient bile into the gut.

"Why am I not producing enough bile?"

Great question, Isla! For Isla, we will soon discover she had some significant liver and detoxification issues. Bile is produced in the liver, which is then stored in the gallbladder, ready to squirt into the intestines when you eat food. If the liver is struggling, bile production can be put on the back-burner. It can also lead to sludgy bile and gallstones, making it even more difficult to secrete bile when you need it to breakdown fat in food. Bile issues can lead to things like nausea, reflux, bloating, diarrhoea as well as non gut-related symptoms, like hormonal imbalances.

"The thing is, Isla, your body *needs* fat in order to produce hormones."

"But I eat plenty of fat," Isla said. "I'm mostly keto." (Ahh, the good old keto diet - we'll get to that one later).

"Eating fat is all good and well. But if you're not producing enough bile to actually breakdown and absorb the fat into your cells, then you may as well be eating none!"

Isla folded her arms. "Right, ok," she slowly nodded. "So I'm not breaking down food in my gut very well, and that's causing more hormone issues?"

Connecting the dots, I like it.

But hormonal issues weren't the only thing Isla was struggling with. She also suffered from anxiety.

"While we're on the topic of the gut," Isla continued. "The weird thing is, when I have an anxiety attack, I also get reflux."

"Is it also accompanied with chest tightness or upper back pain, and feeling like you can't breathe?" I asked.

"Yes! But actually, I never feel like I can breathe deeply."

"Let me tell you about hiatal hernia, Isla. Get ready to have your socks knocked off!"

A hiatal hernia is also a dysfunction that impacts your digestive organs. A hiatal hernia occurs when your stomach wedges up through the diaphragm wall, into your oesophagus. It can stay up there for good, or it can slide up and down, depending on what state you're in. It sounds pretty nasty, but it's extremely common. In fact, it has been found that over 40% of the western population has a sliding hiatal hernia. If your stomach is partly stuck up in your oesophagus, it can make breaking down foods really difficult. A common symptom is reflux, as the food regurgitates back into your oesophagus. Plus your stomach acid production reduces when you have a hiatal hernia, making it even harder to breakdown foods.

"Ok, right, so that makes sense about the reflux. But what does my stomach have to do with my anxiety attacks?" Isla asked.

"So much, Isla, so much."

You see, when the stomach wedges up into the oesophagus, your stomach also presses onto your heart and your lungs. It can lead to feelings of chest tightness, palpitations, and inability to breathe. And because your organs are wedged together, it can also cause chest and upper back pain.

"Sounds a lot like an anxiety attack, hey?"

Isla shook her head, her mouth gaped open. "Are you serious? I'm getting anxiety attacks because of my stomach? Place your hands on me Filly, and fix it!" Isla cried. "Do I need to fly down to your clinic?"

For local clients, I would usually test and treat the hiatal hernia myself in our clinic. But fortunately for patients interstate, we have at-home instructionals to effectively self-treat a hiatal hernia. It's incredibly easy to do, and can make a world of difference.

There are many other ways GI organs can breakdown. Alongside bile and stomach acid production issues, your pancreas can fail to produce adequate digestive enzymes to further breakdown foods. Without sufficient nutrients from food, you can imagine how quickly other body systems - like the brain, the adrenals, the mitochondria, the detox pathways - will burnout. One of the major root causes that switch digestive juices off is, wait for it...stress. I see this time and time again with "busy" people on-the-go, doing-doing-doing. When you're in a constant state of fight-or-flight, your nervous system switches off your digestive organs. If this happens chronically, your digestive organs fail to secrete juices effectively. Not chewing your food properly also causes major strain on your digestive organs, causing them to burnout over time (yep, I'm talking to you lady, always eating on the run!).

And finally, I can't talk about the digestive organs without talking about the beautiful creation that is your gut lining. Fun fact: did you know that your intestinal wall, if completely stretched out, is almost the surface area of a football field? What the?! The gut lining has two major roles: to absorb nutrients, and to support immune function.

In regards to absorption, your gut lining contains tight junctions of microvilli (little finger-like projections across the gut lining that absorb nutrients). When it becomes damaged (often due to stress - um, hello again stress! - poor diet, medications, pathogens, toxins), junctions start to separate. This is called intestinal permeability; you might've heard it as "leaky gut." It's a nasty thing to have. Not only can it cause major gut issues (imagine having an open wound 24/7 in your belly!), but it can really screw up your immune system. Every time a piece of undigested food, or nasty stuff like pathogens and toxins, pass through a leaky gut and enters your bloodstream, your immune system stands at attack. These chunky particles are foreign to the body, and the immune system tags them as "dangerous." This immune attack causes a whole lot of inflammation, and has been linked to autoimmune conditions like Hashimotos, Ceoliac Disease, Fibromyalgia and Inflammatory Bowel Disease (IBD). Food allergies and sensitives are also very common with leaky gut.

We test most of these digestive organs using the same stool test that detects pathogens. The beauty about this lab test is that it's picking up functional imbalances. You might've seen your GP already, and had bloods taken and maybe an X-ray or ultrasound of your abdomen. While these tests can pick up gallstones, bowel obstruction and structural abnormalities, they aren't sensitive enough to pick up functional imbalances like the production of digestive juices, leaky gut or how well your immune system is functioning within your gut lining. Colonoscopies and endoscopies are also medical tests routinely used, but these tests are used mostly to diagnose diseases like IBD and bowel cancer. A hiatal hernia can also be diagnosed with an endoscopy, but it will only be detected if it's bigger than 2cm - the smaller ones go undiagnosed, yet continue to cause major strife.

Hazel (coming up next), had all the GP and gastroenterologist gut tests, only to be brushed-off by her doctor that everything looked fine. "You just have Irritable Bowel Syndrome," her doc had said. "You'll have to learn to deal with it - just be careful with what you eat".

Microbiome/SIBO - hey Hazel, hey

"I'm fed-up," Hazel said, slamming a hand on the table. "I can't even eat flaming bananas anymore. Even garlic gives me the runs! It feels like I'm reacting to everything, and not just junk food. I'm even nervous to be away from the toilet. Can you believe it, I actually almost shat my pants the other day? And my doctor says I have to learn to deal with it?"

Hazel's big body burnout issue was her gut, and it was no surprise, when we did testing, that her microbiome was dysbiotic. Hazel had it in her head that her bloating and "crazy" bowel movements (urgent loose stools one day, constipation the next) all came down to food allergies.

"Why do you think that?" I asked Hazel.

"Because every time I eat, my gut flares up. I can't work out what foods are doing it. I might eat, say, a banana one day and be ok, but the next it causes instant bloating. Can I just do a food allergy test? I'm sick of trying to figure it all out."

"Yes, we can. But even if you are showing food sensitivities, my big question would be *why?* I don't believe you should live on a restricted diet forever. Food sensitivities almost always come back to an imbalanced gut."

Enter: the microbiome.

The microbiome is the centre of it all. The empire of your health. In recent times, there has been a plethora of research linking good health (and not so good health) to the state of your microbiome. The microbiome compromises trillions of bacterial, fungal, viral and protozoa microbes. If your microbiome is healthy, you will have a good amount of beneficial bacteria, like bifidobacterium species, lactobacillus species, akkermansia muciniphila and faecalibacterium prausnitzii (try to say those ten times!). These lovely lads help you to break down food to a useable form, support the gut lining and regular bowel movements, produce anti-inflammatory metabolic by-products, and make up a large chunk of your immune system.

The rest of your microbiome will be made up of commensal bacteria, fungi and viral microbes. These commensal microbes are healthy and beneficial in small amounts, but they are also opportunistic and can easily overgrow when given the right circumstances (i.e. antibiotic use, processed diet, eating too fast, alcohol, stress, lack of sleep, and toxins). As opportunistic microbes overgrow, they squash out the beneficial microbes. This becomes a recipe for disaster. Not only do you lose all the anti-inflammatory and immune-boosting effects of the good bugs, but on top of this, the opportunistic microbes contain lipopolysaccharide (LPS) in their cell walls, which trigger an inflammatory response when bacterial levels get too high.

"So you're saying you think my microbiome is screwed up, and that's causing my food sensitivities?" Hazel asked, drumming her perfectly manicured fingernails on the table.

"Possibly. But let me ask you a few questions first. When exactly does the bloating happen? Is it like, 15-30 minutes after eating? Or is it more like an hour or two later?"

Hazel's drumming fingernails stopped. "Oh, definitely within 15-30 minutes."

"Gotcha. Let me tell you about SIBO."

Overgrowth of microbes can occur in both the large intestines and the small intestines. Overgrowth that occurs in the small intestines, is known as small intestinal bacterial overgrowth, or SIBO. Clinically, I have seen far more intensive gut issues when a patient has SIBO, in comparison to large intestinal bacterial overgrowth. Why? Because, unlike in the large intestines, high amounts of bacteria should *not* be living in the small intestines. Every time you eat food, your gut muscles *should* contract, and push food through the small intestines, sweeping out any lingering bacteria from the small intestines, into the large intestines where food gets munched up and fermented by the army of microbes waiting below. This contraction of muscles is called your gastrointestinal motility. When this sweeping, cleaning action between each meal doesn't occur appropriately, bacteria can take up camp in the small intestines. Compromised motility is a common cause of SIBO. Other causes include chronic antibiotic use, food poisoning, abdominal surgery, compromised digestive juices, medications and stress.

"Right, so I might have some bugs hanging in my small intestines. But what's the big deal?" Hazel asked. I could tell by the narrowing of her eyes that she wasn't 100% sold on the idea of SIBO causing her food reactions.

"The big deal? So much! In fact, you know how your doctor labelled you with IBS? Well, emerging research shows that up to 85% of mysterious 'IBS' cases are actually SIBO cases."

Hazel's eyes perked up. "Ok, tell me more."

When bacteria is stuck in the small intestines, they start feeding and fermenting on food in the small intestines - in the *wrong* area of the gut. Fermentation causes gas. It's normal if it occurs in your large intestines. You'll just fart it out. But when it occurs in the small intestines, the gas, in the wrong area, causes your gut to blow up like a balloon, causing bloating and painful distention. This can then disrupt bowel movements, as food and faecal matter struggle to move from one end of your gut to the other. And, it can make you feel like you're having all sorts of food reactions, which is why many people with SIBO believe their gut issues are all food sensitivity related.

Hazel placed a hand over her mouth, and started nodding. "Ok, ok." I could see the lights switch on in her eyes.

"But bloating is not the only issue with SIBO," I continued. "It can also start affecting other body systems."

"What, like affecting my stress and energy levels?"

"Exactly!"

SIBO can lead to nutrient deficiencies. You absorb up to 95% of nutrients in the small intestines. If you've got a bunch of bacteria stuck in the small intestines, it can compromise your ability to absorb nutrients. Plus, SIBO is also very inflammatory and can tear away at the gut lining and break down brush border enzymes in your intestinal tract, making it even more difficult to absorb nutrients. This then affects the neuroendocrine and detox systems, which can cause things like, yep, you guessed it - anxiety and fatigue. I commonly see skin issues like rashes, dermatitis, rosacea and acne with SIBO also.

"Well give me a test, woman!" Hazel blurted.

I laughed at her no-nonsense attitude. "You're speaking my language, Hazel. Test not guess!"

Because Hazel didn't want to stuff around, she did a comprehensive stool test to look at pathogens, GI organs and the microbiome in the large intestinal tract. And to ensure we didn't miss anything, we also chucked in a SIBO test from Nutripath (check out Appendix for more info). SIBO is tested by measuring bacterial gas levels in the small intestines via breath. Sure enough, Hazel's SIBO markers were through the roof. Her stool test also showed leaky gut, digestive enzyme deficiencies, and depleted beneficial microbiome.

"I just can't believe I did all those tests with the gastroenterologist," Hazel said. "I even let him stick a camera up my bum! And they didn't find any of this."

And that, my friend, is why I love functional medicine lab testing.

Vaginal ecosystem - Rose's lady parts

Lovely Rose and her lovely vagina. Well, it didn't feel so lovely when she first started working with us. Rose was struggling big time with what she thought was thrush (aka candida overgrowth). And initially, that made a lot of sense, seeing as though her stool test showed candida overgrowth in the gut. But her vaginal issues went deeper than fungi in her lady parts.

Like the gut, the vagina has an amazing ecosystem of microbes - mostly bacteria and yeast microbes. In perfect balance, the vaginal ecosystem will carry on happily. But, like the gut, opportunistic bacteria and yeast can easily overgrow, which can lead to vaginal issues like itchiness, funky discharge, smelliness, broken, irritated skin, and discomfort, especially during sex. Because these opportunistic microbes spit out inflammatory metabolites, they can also affect your energy, mood, hormones, sex-drive and even cause infertility. The vaginal ecosystem becomes disrupted in very similar ways to that of the gut microbiome: antibiotics, stress, suppressed immune system, and a processed diet heavy in refined carbs and sugar (hello again sugar, Rose!). In addition, using diaphragms, increased frequency of sex, spermicides and vaginal douching/washing can also cause vaginal ecosystem dysbiosis.

Along with her fatigue and low mood, Rose was also struggling with vaginal issues. It all started around the same time her body crashed with exhaustion post glandular-fever and having babies. Her vagina was constantly itchy, and she often found stinky discharge in her undies. It would get worse with ovulation and leading up to her period. Any libido she had lingering, was squashed every time the vaginal infection flared up.

"My poor husband. Between my exhaustion, low mood, and my annoying vagina - there's no chance for us," Rose had said, dropping her head in her hands, deflated. "I just feel so yuck all the time. And the itch. It's enough to drive anyone insane!"

Before coming to see us, Rose had tried addressing (what she thought was) thrush with anti-fungal creams and suppositories. They helped for a bit, but the "thrush" kept coming back.

"Do you know if it's actually thrush?" I asked Rose.

"Well I haven't had it tested. But what I read on Google, it sounds like thrush. It's cottage-cheese looking most of the time, and smells a bit yeasty."

"Most of the time?"

"Well, sometimes the discharge is more runny, and a bit yellow or green. And it can smell a bit..." She looked around, trying to find the word.

"Fishy?"

"Yes!"

"Ok," I said. "You might not have thrush. Or if you do, you might also have a bacterial infection."

Rose wasn't alone. Most women immediately assume they have thrush when they start to get itchy in their vagina. They try to treat the infection with anti-fungals. But bacterial infections, often referred to as bacterial vaginosis, are also incredibly common. If you're treating the infection using anti-fungals, when actually it is a bacterial infection, you can make the bacterial infection worse as anti-fungals create a more alkaline environment (your vagina should be very acidic), which can cause a further overgrowth of opportunistic bacteria that thrive in a more alkaline environment. If you have both infections, most women will find a relief using anti-fungals, but the itchiness and discharge continues coming back, because the bacterial infection is never addressed. And let's just say you also have a sexually transmitted infection (STI) added to the mix, well the more dysbiotic your vaginal microbiome, the more the STI will flare up.

If a patient is experiencing a once-off acute vaginal infection, I would usually suggest doing a quick vaginal pH swab test. These can be easily picked up from the chemist or online, usually for around 15 dollars. As I mentioned earlier, the vagina should be very acidic. If the swab remains yellow, it is more likely that you have a candida issue, because candida can live in an acidic environment. But if the swab changes to a blue or green colour, triggered by a high pH (alkaline) reading, then it is more likely you have a pathogenic bacterial infection.

For Rose, however, because of her chronic vaginal issues, I wanted to look deeper into her vaginal ecosystem. And so we ran a comprehensive vaginal microbiome profile swab test, which detects not just pH levels, but also identifies specific pathogenic bacteria and yeast microbes, and STI's. And unlike a general vaginal swab that you might do with your GP, the functional vaginal swab test also looks at the health of the vaginal beneficial bacteria, which is *absolutely critical* for a happy, thriving vagina.

Rose did her test, and, surprise, surprise, she had more going on than just thrush. Yes, candida levels were very high, but she also had bacterial vaginosis, a high pH (alkaline) reading, and her beneficial bugs were below detectable limits. No wonder she couldn't clear up the ongoing vaginal infection - her good bugs, the bugs that help modulate a healthy, balanced ecosystem, had conked out.

"I wish I'd come to see you guys years ago," Rose cried.

We hear this all the time. So much unnecessary suffering that could be prevented.

Throughout this chapter, you have seen through the experiences of Hazel, Rose and Isla, how imbalances in these areas can lead to body burnout symptoms (and not just gut symptoms, but so much more!), and how you can test these areas to confirm imbalances. You've also discovered some root causes, that cause the GI system to burnout in the first place. We'll dive deeper into these, later in the book.

Coming up next, is the third and last body system: the detoxification system.

SUMMARY
GASTROINTESTINAL SYSTEM

In this chapter, you have learned about the body systems that make up the GI system:

Pathogens	**Digestive Organs**
Parasites, worms, bacterial, viral and yeast pathogens	The stomach, the pancreas, the gall bladder and the gut lining
Microbiome / SIBO	**Vaginal Ecosystem**
Your beneficial bacteria, and when the bacteria overgrows into the small intestines	Thrush, bacterial vaginosis, sexually transmitted diseases and your good vaginal bacteria

CHAPTER 3

Detoxification System

```
Detox          |  Methylation
---------------+---------------
Oxidation/     |  Nutrient
Inflammation   |  Replacement
```

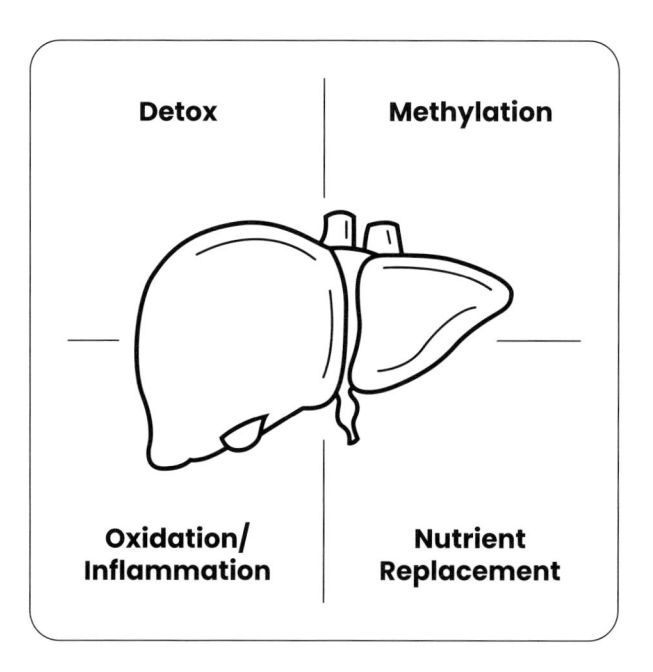

Introduction

If you thought the gut was cool, just wait until we go through the detoxification system. In this chapter, you'll learn all about the four main areas that make up the detox system - detox pathways, methylation, oxidation/inflammation and nutrient replacement. The organs involved in the detox system are the liver, the kidneys, the lymphatic system, as well as the elimination pathways (the pipes/holes you wee, poop and sweat out of).

While many health gurus tout the gut as being the "centre" of all health, I would argue the detox system is just as important (some might even argue *more* important). Why? Because one of the major roles of the detox system is to break down nasty toxins and clear them from the body. When the detox system stops working properly, toxins will build up in your system, and basically poison you from the inside out - yuck! The detox system also helps to convert nutrients into a usable form, metabolise hormones, and burn fat. It's incredibly important for so many things.

In this chapter, you'll get a clear understanding of the areas in the detox system, why they're important, how they burnout, and how to know if your detox system needs some investigating.

Detox pathways - Toxic Isla

Isla was feeling "toxic." She didn't use that term. But I could see from her symptom presentation *and* her lifestyle, that something was up with the detox pathways - or at least I was highly suss about it.

"What do you do for work, Isla?"

"I run a hair salon. I've been a hairdresser for the past 25 years," she said, smoothing her blonde hair with her hand. Isla was the type of lady that looked like she was going out for a night on the town - *everyday,* even when she was going to the gym.

"That's a lot of chemical exposure," I said, matter-of-factly, without judgement.

"Yeah, I guess. The dyes and commercial cleaning stuff can give me a headache sometimes - at least I think that's what it is."

"Really? Ok." Note to self: chemical sensitivity.

Isla, as we saw earlier, was struggling with hormone issues, weight gain and anxiety. She was also really struggling with sleep.

"It's crazy. I wake up at 2am every morning without fail. It's been going on for years. And sometimes I can't get back to sleep. And nightmares, I have so many nightmares."

Waking up in the early hours. Nightmares. This is commonly seen in people with detox issues, as the liver works hardest between the hours of 1am-5am. If the liver is already struggling, it can be a "stressful" experience trying to clear toxins through your detox pathways. This extra stress can literally wake you up at night.

The sleep issues. Oestrogen excess. Weight gain. Bile production issues. High exposure to toxins. Chemical-triggered headaches. Oh, and a lover of wine and bubbles. It was all pointing to detox issues for Isla.

Detox refers to how well your liver and eliminatory pathways (i.e. lymph, kidneys, bile) are working. Detoxification works on three phases. Phase 1 and 2 occur in the liver. Phase 1 converts fat soluble toxins into water soluble toxins, and requires a hefty amount of antioxidants (like vitamins A, B's, C, D, E and CoQ10) to do so. The liver then passes the toxins over to phase 2 liver detox, which breaks down toxins, ready for excretion. You need a good amount of sulfur containing amino acids (like glutathione, glycine, n-acetylcysteine, l-arginine) for phase 2 to function. Once toxins are broken down, they're then expelled from the body (phase 3 detox) through your faeces, urine and sweat.

"Ok, right," Isla said. "Well how do these phases burnout? Is it really all to do with me just being a hairdresser?"

"Being exposed to high levels of chemicals will certainly put more stress on your liver and burn through required nutrients needed to detoxify properly, but there are likely other causes at play."

When I did my own urine test to examine my detox pathways using an organic acids test (yep, the same one that also measures the brain and mitochondria), I was shocked to see how burned-out my pathways were. I'd been living a low-tox life for several years prior to testing. I'd been eating a low-processed diet. I'd gotten on the DIY band-wagon, ditching all the toxic cleaning and skincare products from my home, and making my own products with natural ingredients. Heck, I hadn't even drunk alcohol or coffee or smoked cigarettes! So why were my detox pathways taxed?

The fact of the matter is that our world is more toxic than ever. In her book, *Low Tox Life*, Alexx Stuart prefers to use the term "low tox" as we can never live 100% free of toxins (at least in my lifetime, anyway!). Plus I had been living almost three decades prior to "cleaning up my toxic-act," using chemical-laden products, eating processed foods, breathing in petrol fumes, drinking chlorinated water, being exposed to electricity, and growing up (and working in) a flower farm where pesticides were regularly sprayed right near our house. Sometimes the damage done to the detox pathways don't just "bounce back" on their own when you start to live low-tox, and therapeutic intervention is needed.

"But gut issues can also compromise the detox pathways," I said to Isla. "Remember we saw that marker on your stool test, showing bacterial overgrowth that was clinging onto your oestrogen and recirculating it back into your system, rather than pooing the excess oestrogen out?"

"Yep, I do."

"Well those bacteria cling onto toxins once they are dumped back into the gut ready for excretion, as well. So yes, you have more chemical exposure compared to the next person, because of your profession. But your gut issues will also be compromising your detox pathways. Not only are you *not* clearing toxins effectively via your bowels, but you're also recirculating those toxins back to your liver, putting a further burden on the liver. And to make matters worse, if you're not breaking down and absorbing nutrients properly in the gut, then your detox pathways won't have the antioxidants and amino acids they need to function optimally."

Isla nodded slowly. I could see her mind ticking over. It's all connected…It's all connected.

"And to go one step further," I continued. "If you've got nervous system issues, like anxiety, it's going to switch your gut off from functioning properly, which can lead to pathogen overgrowth in the first place."

"Right, so my detox issues might be caused by my anxiety?"

"One cause, yes. There are often many sticky root causes. We'll get to those soon enough!"

Isla had previously had a full blood count with her GP. They had checked her liver enzymes, which all came back fine. Crazily enough when we did Isla's organic acids test, her detox pathways were pretty burned-out, especially her glutathione stores.

"I don't get it. Why are your tests showing I have liver issues, but my GP tests didn't?"

Such a common question. The reason for this is that GP liver function tests look more specifically at liver enzymes dying off, which are signs of fatty liver disease. Our functional lab tests look at all the different pathways, as well as specific nutrient markers that can pinpoint where in the detox pathways things have gone wrong. Some of our worst detox patient cases, have had "perfect" GP liver function test results.

Methylation - Rose's mutated genes

Another issue that can really stuff up your detoxification system is genetic mutations. One of the most common genetic mutations that can affect your ability to detoxify is a mutation in methylation, or methylenetetrahydrofolate reductase (MTHFR). MTHFR is an enzyme that breaks down the amino acid homocysteine. It's very important for removing toxins from the body, repairing DNA, keeping inflammation in check, and keeping your myelin (protective coating around the nerves) healthy. When MTHFR mutates, these functions can become severely compromised, and it also affects the way you utilise and metabolise certain nutrients, in particular vitamin B12 and folate.

"MTHFR, I'm so sure I have this!" Rose exclaimed, when we were going over her health history and body systems in her initial consult. She pulled out some tattered test results from her handbag, and started flicking through the pages. "There!" She pointed at a marker. "There, it says there that I have the MTHFR mutated genes."

I picked up the papers. Rose had done an online gene test. I'm not a fan of buying random lab tests online - there are so many companies out there not doing proper or reliable analyses. I'd prefer to run a MTHFR Gene Mutation test from Nutripath (check out Appendix for more info).

"That's great info to have," I said to Rose. "It can definitely help us to further connect the dots. It could certainly be contributing to your fatigue, brain fog and low mood - these are all common signs of an MTHFR issue."

I often see other inflammatory issues connected with an MTHFR mutation: body aches, headaches, migraines, food sensitivities, hormonal issues, infertility and fluid retention. If the MTHFR gene is completely shut down, it can lead to full-blown mental ill health disorders, like suicidal depression/anxiety, bipolar and schizophrenia.

"But my big question, Rose, is: is your MTHFR mutation expressing?"

"What do you mean? I thought once you have a genetic issue it's always there?"

Well yes, a genetic mutation *is* always there. But it might not be causing any issues. You see, mutated genes will only express if given the right environment. Emotional stress, trauma, inflammatory foods, alcohol, environmental toxins, poor gut health, mould and viral infections can all trigger a genetic mutation to express. And even some people without the MTHFR gene mutation can start experiencing methylation issues, if their body is under a lot of stress and burning through important nutrients that support methylation.

People who discover mutations on genetic tests, can get fixated on these mutations, thinking all their issues stem from that genetic defect. The fact is, not all mutations express.

"It's all good and well to know if you have a genetic issue," I said to Rose. "But what's more valuable to know is if it's actually expressing."

"Ok, that makes sense. Well how can we know?"

Enter the wonderful organic acids test again. This urine test has specific markers that relate to methylation. It can show if your mutated genes are actually acting up.

Rose's test results showed very depleted B12 and folate, which told us that yes, her "dirty genes" (a term coined by Dr Ben Lynch) were expressing. The interesting thing for Rose, however, is that she had felt pretty healthy for most of her life. Symptomatically speaking, the MTHFR mutated gene was likely lying dormant. Until, that is, she started having babies and sleepless nights, as well as the mould exposure and glandular fever infection. This combination of "stressors" most likely switched her mutated MTHFR genes on, which contributed to her body system burnout, and cascade of health symptoms.

Oxidation/inflammation – hot hot Hazel

Hazel was on fire. But not in the "you go girl!" kind of way. Her body was literally inflamed.

"Inflamed – yes! That's how I feel half the time," Hazel cried. "My gut is always on fire. I get hot and itchy all over. My mind feels fried most of the time. What's going on with me?"

Well, as we know, Hazel had some pretty serious adrenal and gut issues. Both these imbalances can cause inflammation. When the adrenals are out of whack, your body becomes very catabolic, meaning it literally starts eating away at tissues and burning up anti-inflammatory nutrients. And an inflamed, angry gut will always cause inflammation in other areas of the body.

When we did lab testing on Hazel's detoxification system, she showed high levels of inflammation in her body, including inflammation of the brain (yep, we could see this!), and oxidative damage at a cellular level. Her stool test also showed inflammation of the bowel, which was likely flaring up overall inflammation levels.

Hazel looked at me, a bit confused. "So you're saying that my messed up gut is inflaming my brain?"

"Yes, that's correct. Have you heard of the gut-brain connection?"

"I've heard of it. But I don't know much about it."

Buckle up for this one, Hazel. So you have a nerve - the vagus nerve - that runs from your brain to your gut. They're constantly sending signals to each other. When your gut is inflamed, it sends inflammatory signals up to the brain, and it can literally leach protective brain nutrients to try and deal with the inflammation in the gut. This then shows up as brain inflammation.

"Is that why I'm not coping with stress like I used to? It feels like every time my gut flares up, so do my stress levels."

Yes ma'am. Hazel was on the money

Inflammation arises due to oxidative stress. Oxidative stress is an imbalance between free radicals (highly reactive chemicals that can damage other cells) and antioxidants in your body. This imbalance will occur when there is a high load of "stressors" causing free radicals to circulate in your body (things like environmental toxins, processed foods, over-exercising, injuries, pathogens, emotional stress), which then causes you to burn through antioxidant nutrients like vitamins A, D, E, CoQ10 and glutathione. It becomes a vicious cycle - the more the inflammatory stressors, the more your antioxidant stores get burned up, leading to further inflammation and oxidative damage to your cells.

DETOXIFICATION SYSTEM

"Right, so my gut and other stuff going on inside my body is likely causing more inflammation?" Hazel asked.

"Yep, and the more inflamed other areas become, the deeper the cellular damage, and the more symptomatic you become."

"Makes sense why I'm feeling so crappy!"

While many people come to us when they are feeling symptomatic and in pain, preventative medicine has always been at the heart of functional medicine. Picking up on oxidative damage and inflammation imbalances can literally save your life. Not just save you from inflammatory symptoms like fatigue, anxiety, bloating, body aches, headaches, allergies, and the like. But save you from terminal illnesses like cancer. Almost all patients we have worked with who have had cancer, have had extremely high levels of inflammation.

You don't want to get to that point. Test. Treat. Restore. Prevent. And live a beautiful, long and healthy life.

Nutrient replacement - Isla and her nails

"I have white spots all over my nails," Isla said, holding up her manicured, polished red nails to the computer screen. "I know you can't see them, because of the polish. But they're riddled with white spots. It's so ugly!"

"That's a common sign of zinc and/or calcium deficiency," I said.

Nutrient replacement makes up the last square in the detoxification system. It's the final piece of all the body systems - and it's not just specific to the detox system. The reason why it's the final piece, is because nutrient deficiencies will only manifest, due to imbalances in one or more of the body systems. For example, if you're in adrenal fatigue, and in a catabolic state, you'll burn through antioxidant minerals and vitamins like magnesium and vitamin C. Or if your gut isn't breaking down foods properly due to GI organ breakdown or pathogenic overgrowth, you can become deficient in literally *any* nutrient. It's common to see iron deficiency in this case. And if your detox pathways are in a state of burnout, or genetic issues are expressing, you'll rapidly burn up nutrients like glutathione and vitamin B's.

Address the imbalances in the body systems first, *then* replace the missing nutrients.

This is the complete reversal of what you will experience if you go to a GP. They'll run a few nutrient panels, usually vitamin D, B12 and iron. And if any of these nutrients are deficient they'll likely tell you to take a supplement or have an infusion. There is rarely any investigation into why you're deficient in the first place. If you have a more holistic GP, they might tell you to go sit in the sun, or eat more red meat. The crazy thing is, many patients who have been given this advice, are already getting enough sun and nutrients from food - yet they still show up with nutritional deficiencies time and time again.

"Yes, this happened to me!" Isla said. "I kept showing up with low iron. I upped my red meat. I even got some iron infusions. Yet my iron continued to show up low. All my GP said was keep taking an iron supplement."

This will never address the root cause.

Address the body system imbalances, address the root causes, *then* (if needed), build deficient nutrient stores back up with targeted supplements and foods.

Oh, and by the way, GP testing for vitamins D, B12 and iron are only three of hundreds of nutrients that make up and support a healthy body. If I want to get a really deep insight into a patient's nutrient status, I will run a blood and urine test - NutriStat from Nutripath (check out Appendix for more info) - that look at all your minerals, vitamins, amino acids and fatty acids.

Just like Isla's white spots on her nails, here are some common visual signs that you might be nutrient deficient (but remember, don't jump to supplementing first - test and treat the underlying cause, then supplement if needed):

- White spots on nails - zinc, calcium deficiency
- Bleeding gums and slow-healing wounds - vitamin C deficiency
- Brittle hair and nails - biotin deficiency
- Mouth ulcers and cracks at sides of the mouth - vitamin B12 deficiency
- Poor night vision and white growth on the eyes - vitamin A deficiency

- Muscle cramping and restless legs - magnesium deficiency
- Hair loss, dizziness, fatigue - low iron.

Throughout this chapter, you have seen through the experiences of the three women, how imbalances in these areas can lead to body burnout symptoms (and even full-blown diseases like cancer), and how you can test these areas to confirm imbalances. You've also discovered some root causes, that cause the detox system to burnout in the first place.

Now you know what body systems are causing which symptoms, the big question is: what causes these body systems to burn out in the first place? What are the deeper root-causes? And how can we restore the body back to good health, for good? The following parts of this book will dive deeper into the root-causes, especially as they apply to Rose, Hazel and Isla. We will look into the mind, habits that support the body, and environmental root-causes (as shown in figure 3.1).

To start the investigation, we have to go right back to the origin of body burnout: the mind.

Figure 3.1: Root-Cause Matrix

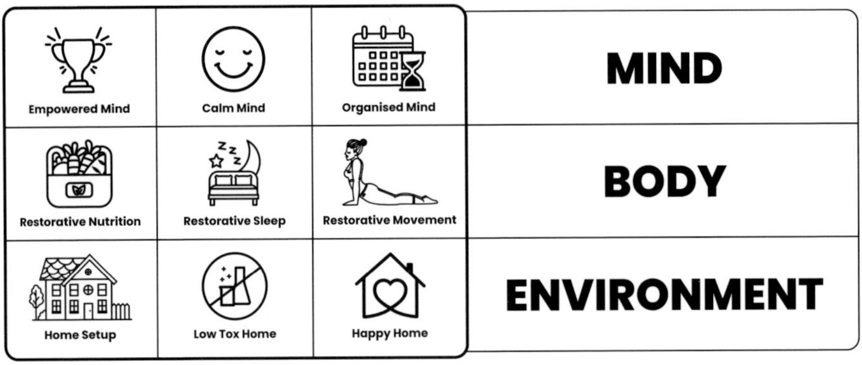

Empowered Mind	Calm Mind	Organised Mind	**MIND**
Restorative Nutrition	Restorative Sleep	Restorative Movement	**BODY**
Home Setup	Low Tox Home	Happy Home	**ENVIRONMENT**

SUMMARY
DETOXIFICATION SYSTEM

In this chapter, you have learned about the parts that make up the detoxification system:

Detox Pathways
The three phases of detoxing, involving the liver and elimination pathways

Methylation
An important enzyme that removes toxins from the body, repairs DNA, and keeps inflammation in check, and that is commonly mutated

Oxidation / Inflammation
How inflammation in the body arises due to oxidative stress

Nutrient Replacement
How nutrient deficiencies arise when the other body systems are out-of-whack

---

Scan to do scorecard

If you haven't done so already, take our **Ending Body Burnout Assessment** - http://chrisandfilly.fm/scorecard. It will pinpoint the main contributors of body burnout that we are about to cover.

STEP TWO
Heal Thy Mind

STEP TWO
HEAL THY MIND

In Step Two, I go over the next step for ending your body burnout for good, and that is healing the mind.

The mind? You say. *Are you serious? You think I'm exhausted and PMS-y and bloated and in pain because I thought myself sick?*

But I "do" mindfulness and meditate. My mind is fine!

I've seen a psychologist and I'm still sick. My body burnout symptoms have nothing to do with my mind.

I just need to do testing and take some supplements and change my diet and sleep more, then I'll get better. I don't need to "heal" my mind.

These are common objections we hear time and time again when we suggest that at the deepest root-cause of body burnout for "busy" people juggling all the things is the mind.

To be honest, I felt the same way when I started my own healing journey. I felt pain in my body and so I thought it was a "physical" problem. Even the anxiety, I felt was due to a depleted body post-births. And so I went seeking solutions to heal my body. I changed my diet, my sleeping patterns, my exercise regime, and ditched toxic chemicals from the home. I did all the lab tests, took all the supplements. I even added in stress-management techniques like breathing exercises and "managed" my time. I stopped running around like a chook without her head, saying "yes" to everyone and everything, hustling and grinding, and working "hard." At the time, this was enough to heal my body (at least initially). The anxiety eased, the heartburn disappeared, the chronic back pain improved, I stopped catching all the colds and flus, the chemical sensitivities cleared up, my cycle was regular, the PMS was mostly non-existent, and my skin was so much better. I was close to being pretty much symptom-free. I was elated - I had healed! But, if I'm really honest, deep down I still had felt "fragile." I felt like I had to wrap myself up in bubble-wrap so I could "manage" and stay on top of my health. I had to eat perfectly, I had to get nine hours of sleep at night, I had to stop exercising intensely, I needed a lot of time away from the kids. If I didn't get any of these, symptoms would start erupting.

Then the COVID-19 pandemic hit in 2020, and my whole world tilted. Our other business, a gym, shutdown. We had to pivot my health practice to become online, and provide the bulk of our income. There was homeschooling while working. We were struggling financially. Then there was the whole emotional upheaval of lockdowns, border closures, vaccine mandates, and feeling like I was in the middle of a witch-hunt! I'd never experienced sleep issues before, but all of a sudden I started developing patterns of insomnia. Then anxiety flared-up. So did back pain, and acne, and hormone imbalances, low-immunity, and heartburn. Some of the symptoms settled over-time, but they were very much simmering beneath the surface, and despite my best efforts to address the lingering symptoms with the same physical healing protocols I had used five years earlier, I couldn't quite get on top of some of the issues, especially the heartburn and almost daily chest tightness and feelings of anxiousness.

I knew there was something deeper I needed to heal. Something hidden. Something stuck in my mind and my unconscious state. Something that was stressing my nervous system and not allowing my body systems to rebalance fully and wholly. And so I dove into healing my mind and the deep-seated and hidden dysfunctional beliefs I had about myself which were causing 24/7 stress. I hired a coach, Jaemin Frazer, one of Australia's top life coaches and known as the "Insecurity Guy," to help me work through all my unprocessed internal beliefs. (And credit does need to go to Jaemin for many of the concepts in the next Empowered Mind chapter).

Doing inner-work was a game changer. The work wasn't about "behaviour management." I'd done that in the past, I was really good at "doing things" and sticking to a plan, but that wasn't helping. The work involved getting to the deepest fear I had about myself, a belief I created as a child, that deep down I was "weak and incapable." This early belief set up patterns of anxiousness as a child, and then addicted doing into my teens and adult life, as I tried to prove my worth, and be accepted by others. If I could achieve more, I would be more, which meant I would never be exposed as being inherently weak and incapable. But in the end, this dysfunctional behaviour led to my body burnout, and was not allowing me to fully heal.

It wasn't the kids that made me sick, or even the pandemic – these were just the catalysts that further wired my already stressed-out nervous system and wounded unconscious mind. And until I could truly resolve my dysfunctional beliefs about myself, I could never achieve true health and abundance in my life, or even in my relationships, finances, business or spirituality. All the diets and supplements and lifestyle modifications, while they could – and all did – help, there wasn't complete resolution until I healed my mind and re-established rapport with myself.

I won't lie. It was hard work. In fact, only a small percentage of the population actually do this deep, inner healing. Most people don't have the courage to face peering inside themselves, for fear of what they might find, or for fear that they're not cut out to do the deeper healing work. I put it off, too. I tried to do all the physical, surface-level stuff. But my health soon unravelled again. So dear reader, if you truly want to end your body burnout – and I mean *end it*, for good – you cannot skip this step. If you skip straight to healing your body and/or environment, you'll only end up getting short-term improvements, if that.

In Step Two: Heal Thy Mind, you will discover the three important processes when it comes to healing the mind: unlocking your internal power, mastering a calm mind, and becoming clear and organised around what you need to do to heal and reach true health.

CHAPTER 4

Empowered Mind

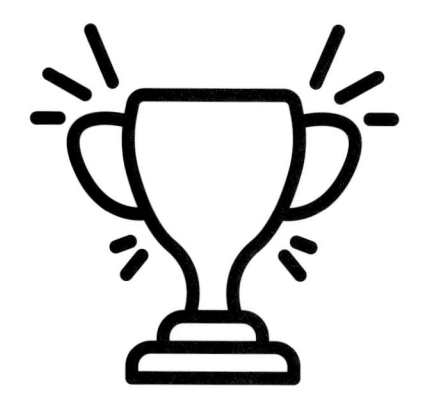

Introduction

In this chapter, you'll learn what you need to do to unlock your own internal power, rewire your brain, and create new empowering beliefs, so you can do the things you need to do to heal from body burnout with self-love and flow, rather than with force and fear. That is what I call *ending* body burnout. I truly believe this is possible.

Without addressing dysfunctional beliefs about yourself, you will never be able to achieve true health. If you're constantly hating on yourself, feeling shame, guilt or thoughts of "I'm not enough," "I'm broken," "I'll never heal," or you're constantly trying to prove your worth, seeking validation or acceptance, or on the defence all the time, your body will remain in a state of stress. The body and mind are connected. What you believe about yourself, will *always* affect your body.

Disempowering beliefs about yourself often show in these ways:

- Emotional eating, staying up late watching Netflix, thrashing your body with exercise (or not exercising at all).
- Constant feelings of negativity, anger, frustration (towards others, especially your family, or yourself), which taxes your adrenals and neurotransmitters.
- Giving up on your health goals too early, or struggling to implement a treatment plan.
- Over-doing and over-working.
- Forcing your way to good health, over-preoccupied with doing everything "right."
- Holding onto trauma or emotionally-charged events, and the stories you have created about yourself based on these experiences, which get stuck in your unconscious state and in your body's tissues, making it difficult - if not impossible - to heal.

In this chapter, you will discover how having a disempowered mind can be at the root-cause of body burnout. You will also discover how you can identify self-limiting beliefs that have led you to where you are now, and how to create a strong enough vision that will propel you forward with unstoppable motivation to heal your body systems at a root-cause level, even when things get tough.

Stuck in motherhood martyrdom - Rose's story

Now, remember, Rose was struggling with exhaustion, brain fog, low mood and sugar-cravings. We discovered in the previous section, that Rose's lab tests showed she had mitochondrial issues, depleted dopamine, candida overgrowth, parasites, low microbiome and methylation issues. But what are the root-causes? What *caused* Rose's body systems to burnout in the first place, and/or preventing her from healing?

Rose was adamant the root-cause was contracting glandular fever, combined with having babies. "That's when my health fell apart, so that must be where it all started," Rose said, with a short, sharp nod.

"Do you think they're the only contributors?" I asked.

"Well, I guess it could be my diet too. You know I can't stop eating sugar, even though I hate myself for it. And maybe I could be going to bed earlier."

"And that's all, they're the root-causes?"

Rose looked at me, blankly, and shrugged.

Rose was stuck in, what I call, motherhood martyrdom. She was the type of mum that did everything for her kids and partner, always leaving herself until last. She was the type of mum who made the perfect school lunchboxes, but then would forget to eat breakfast and lunch herself, and end up bingeing out on biscuits and chocolate in the afternoon. The type of mum who did all the cleaning and the cooking and even the yard work, and then went to work in her business, serving client after client.

"Do you think it might also have something to do with always doing everything for everyone else?" I asked, gently.

Rose sighed. Her face dropped. She suddenly looked ten years older. "You're probably right," Rose said. "So that's the root-cause?"

"It certainly would be causing stress on your system in so many ways. It's doing no favours in allowing your body to heal from the glandular fever and the three close pregnancies. It most likely set your system up to be more susceptible to picking up infections, as well as pregnancy depletion." I paused, to let Rose take all that in. "But Rose," I said. "Is that the root-cause?"

Rose's forehead furrowed. "I'm guessing from your question...no?"

"*Why* are you doing everything for everyone else?"

It turned out that Rose's motherhood martyrdom programming wasn't simply an obligation to care of her kids or her husband or even her clients. Rose's over-caring went right back to her own childhood. Rose described her mother as "aloof." Her

EMPOWERED MIND

mother looked after her, fed her, but emotionally she was absent. Rose had felt like her mother hadn't loved her. And because of this, she had started to believe that maybe there was something wrong with her. If her own mother couldn't love her, the one person who *should've* given her that love, then there must've been something wrong with her - she must be inherently "unlovable."

The important point of Rose's belief, her "story," about herself, however, is that Rose *created* this belief. It wasn't her mother's fault, or even the way she was brought up, although these would've contributed to Rose's sense-making. As I learned from Jaemin Frazer in his book *Unhindered*, Rose was 100% responsible for creating this belief about herself. This is a piece that many people miss when doing self-awareness work. Most people assume that the way they are "programmed" is because of the way they were brought up, the experiences that they had when they were young, and that they had no control over the events that happened to them. But this is only half the story. While events are generally outside of a child's control, the child did make the choice to make the event mean something about themselves (i.e. for Rose, she decided to believe that she was unlovable based on how she was making sense of her mother's behaviour). This insight is incredibly important - instead of blaming people or past events, which puts you into a disempowered state, you are able to take full responsibility for your sense-making about yourself, which means you are now able to take responsibility and create a new meaning about yourself. You are now response-able - or able to respond.

This story that Rose had created about herself in her childhood continued into her adult years. Rose swore she would never be like her mum, and so she gave her heart and soul to her family, and all her relationships, to the detriment of her self.

But the thing is, this behaviour wasn't just about avoiding becoming like her mother. At a deeper level, this behaviour stemmed from a desperate need to feel loved. If she could be a loving mother, a doting wife, a devoted massage therapist, then surely this would mean she would finally be loved. The more insecure Rose felt about herself, the more she needed love and validation from others, the more she sank deeper into over-caring and over-doing for others.

At the deepest level, Rose's root-cause was that she felt unlovable. And this is what caused Rose's health to fall apart in the first place. And until Rose could review, deconstruct and create a more empowering story about herself, true healing would be blocked.

Stuck in addicted doing - Hazel's story

I could tell Hazel wanted a quick-fix, from the moment I first met her. She had that impatient look about her. Always tapping a foot on the floor, or fingernails on the table. Constantly checking her watch or her phone, always distracted.

Hazel was struggling with some pretty intense gut issues, heightened stress response, irritability, and dropping energy levels. It was really affecting her productivity at work, and she was constantly feeling like a Dragon Mum. We discovered on her labs that she had adrenal fatigue, SIBO, leaky gut, depleted digestive enzymes, and high levels of inflammation.

"I don't care how many pills I need to take, just give me what I need to get better and let's get it done," she said, waving her hand towards my supplement cabinet.

I laughed. "Don't worry Hazel, you'll get your pills. But if you truly want to end your body burnout for good, that's going to be only one small part of your treatment plan."

"What else do I need to do?"

"We need to get to the root-cause."

Like Rose, Hazel had layers of root-causes. There were some big issues with her habits and her lifestyle (we'll get to those soon), but at the deepest level, Hazel's body burnout was a result of her constant feelings of inadequacy.

When Hazel was a kid, her parents had high-expectations. She felt pressured to get the best grades at school, win all the races in the athletics carnival, and play the piano to perfection. Hazel tried her hardest to please her parents. But nothing she ever did felt good enough. Her feelings of inadequacy drove her to become a high-achiever, a perfectionist, always trying to prove her worth. Later, when her partner left her shortly after the birth of her second child, she felt the same feelings of inadequacy. *It's finally been validated: I'm not good enough.* Hazel threw herself into her work, climbing up the corporate ladder, grinding herself to the bone. She had always thought she worked so hard for her two sons, to give them financial security that their dad would never give them. But when we did inner work with Hazel, it turned out that her addicted-doing, over-working pattern, stemmed from her need to prove her worth, and hide her deep beliefs of inadequacy.

In the end, Hazel's deepest root-cause was not that she was burning the candle at both ends. It was the fact that she felt inadequate, which drove this behaviour in the first place. And until she could create a more empowering belief about her worth, she would never stop addictive-doing, and as a result, destroying her body. All the supplements in the world would not end her body burnout, until she could solve her deepest root-cause.

Stuck in trauma - Isla's story

Isla had a pattern of quitting early on health programs. She said so when we first caught up for our online consult.

"I've tried all the diets and health courses. I've seen some naturopaths. But I struggle to stick to anything. Gahhh, I just love drinking wine and going out for dinner. I'm hoping this time will be different," she said, biting her perfectly manicured thumb.

Isla was struggling with anxiety, insomnia, weight gain, hot flushes and heavy, painful periods. Her labs revealed low serotonin, oestrogen dominance, h.pylori and detox issues.

"Everything I'd done in the past was just based on guesswork. Now that I can see how screwed up my body systems are on these labs, I'm sure I'll stick to your program," Isla said, still biting her nail.

"Are you sure?" I asked. "Even if it means staying off the wine for awhile?"

Isla's mouth screwed up. She didn't look so sure.

"This is an issue," I said. "*This* is a root-cause."

We dug into why Isla struggled to follow through with a health program. On the surface she thought it was because she struggled to give up the things she loved - the champagne, the decadent deserts. Going a bit deeper, she then admitted that she always gave up because it got too hard, or too inconvenient, or too complicated, or too expensive, or too boring, or she didn't have enough time.

"Are these the real issues, Isla? They sound a bit like excuses."

It took some more digging, but we knew we had hit the root, when Isla's guard came down, and she started crying. "I don't think I can be whole. I don't think I'm worth healing."

Isla had been sexually abused as an early teen. We later worked out that this is when Isla's hormones really went out of whack, and when her anxiety engulfed her. Isla was holding onto stories about herself, that she had created to make sense of the abuse - that she was bad, that she was not worthy. These beliefs had started forming, even before she was abused. She had experienced a "normal" upbringing at home. Loving parents, no neglect. But at school she felt like she wasn't as "smart" as the other kids, and felt more comfortable talking and telling stories. She was constantly getting in trouble by her teachers for being a "chatter-box," and distracting the other kids. Even being sent to the principle's office for being disruptive. "Stop being naughty," was a word she heard often, to the point where she started thinking, *maybe there is something wrong with me, maybe I am actually bad*. When the abuse happened, in Isla's young brain, it validated: *yes, there is something wrong with me. I must truly be bad for this to have happened to me.* Even though Isla had done talk-therapy with a psychologist around the sexual abuse, and she felt like she had moved past and let go of the actual event, she was still plagued with self-worth issues.

Adult Isla wasn't suffering with "anxiety" - that was just the symptom. Isla was suffering from a broken relationship with herself. And until Isla could reprogram her self-limiting beliefs, she would continue staying trapped in this trauma-loop, damaging her body systems, giving up early, yo-yo-ing from one diet or health protocol to another, never giving herself a chance to get well, because she believed herself unworthy.

Self-limiting beliefs: the ultimate power suckers

As we can see in the stories above, self-limiting beliefs are always at the root-cause of body burnout. They suck your internal power, put a massive stress on your nervous system (24/7!), set you up with dysfunctional patterns that lead to poor health, and will prevent you from truly healing, and staying well for life. Everything you do is driven by your internal belief-system. Underneath every thought, feeling, action, behaviour and habit lies a belief. The results you have in your life, including your current health state is also dictated by your belief-system. You cannot exist without having a belief about yourself and your existence in this world. It's how we are hard-wired. It's how our brains are programmed. Without a belief-system you would have no substance to think or act or be what makes us human. So the deepest, most entrenched beliefs you have about yourself matter. They really matter.

SELF-LIMITING BELIEFS LOOK LIKE:

- I'm not good enough
- I'm unworthy
- I'm unlovable
- I'm weak
- I'm incapable
- I'm stupid
- I'm dumb
- I'm untrustworthy
- I'm dangerous
- I'm hopeless
- I'm undeserving
- I'm a failure
- I don't belong
- I'm different

Now, you might read these, and identify straight away that "X" is what you believe about yourself. But most people don't, especially adults, and most especially high-achieving people who are very good at getting stuff done and achieving goals. Why? Because as we grow older, we try to protect ourselves from being exposed - we do all we can to live a life that keeps our deepest fears hidden from others, and even from ourselves.

Yet our unconscious state always knows, and it's dictating everything that happens in our thoughts, feelings, behaviours, and yes, the health of our body. If you regularly experience any of these signs (even just one), you have a self-limiting belief holding you back:

- Feeling anxious, worrying, overwhelmed, stressed-out
- Over-doing, addictive doing, workaholic
- Rushing, hurrying
- Easily offended, defensive, taking things personally
- Overreacting, catastrophising
- Domineering, aggressive, guarded
- Needing to be the centre of attention
- Feeling significant/worthy only when others give you praise
- Stuck in victim-mentality
- Struggle to say sorry
- Jealousy, often playing the comparison-game
- Putting other people down, gossiping
- Feeling bitter - towards others, yourself, your lot in life
- Feeling frustrated with yourself and/or others
- Hiding, pretending, playing games, beating around the bush
- Blaming others/things for your lot in life
- Making excuses
- Feeling shame, guilt, apathy, low self-confidence
- Feeling stuck, not progressing with things like health, business, career, finances, relationships.
- Procrastination, easily distracted

If you're reading this, nodding your head, seeing yourself stuck in self-limiting beliefs and/or dysfunctional patterns, you're probably wondering how you can step out of this vicious cycle.

Let me introduce you to dead reckoning. Dead reckoning is an old maritime term used to describe navigating. In order to travel to a destination, you need to know where you're at now, where you want to go, how you got where you currently are, how you're going to get to your destination, and what might stop you from getting there. Let's have a look at each of these steps.

Where am I now?

Abraham Maslow, a famous psychologist, said: "What is necessary to change a person is to change his awareness of himself." Self-awareness needs to occur both in the present, the past and in the future.

Before going into the darkness of the past or the elusive future, you need to become crystal-clear on where you're at now, your present state. In order to make change, you have to feel enough pain to make change. Change is hard. Change is painful. Creating enough pain and discomfort around your current state, so that it outweighs the pain of changing, is essential for moving forwards with the momentum you need to end your body burnout. I've seen many women - including friends - who are suffering immense pain, yet they soldier on living out their same life, brushing off their pain, or getting stuck in victim-mentality, thinking they have no choice to live like this for the rest of their life, because the thought of changing is uncomfortable. This will only ever end in heartbreak. So firstly, step out of pretence and get honest about what your body burnout is costing you.

Then, take back your power. NLP co-founders Richard Bandler and John Grinder created some core presuppositions around our internal operating systems. One such presupposition is: people work perfectly, you are not broken. Yes, that's right! You might *feel* burned-out and broken (that's the language I used when I first fell sick), but you aren't actually broken. What does this actually mean? Essentially, it means that the results you are getting in every area in your life - including your health - are the results you've designed your system to create, and that your behaviour is serving a need and has positive intention. Therefore you're working "perfectly." You might be thinking: *How the heck is feeling fatigued, anxious and bloated an example of working perfectly, Filly?!* Don't worry, I thought that too when I was introduced to this presupposition. But when I broke down my thought-patterns, behaviours and strategies that led to my body burnout in the first place, it made complete sense! I was stuck in an addictive-doing pattern because it was working really well for me - perfectly in fact. Working hard meant I achieved good grades, completed a

PhD, built a business, which then meant I felt like I had "worth" and "significance" by what I could achieve. And certainly I had plenty of people telling me how awesome I was by what I could "do." Over-doing and over-achieving also worked well to hide from my greatest fear of being weak and incapable - the more I could do and achieve, the easier I could hide from being found out. It was a perfect strategy. And actually an act of self-protection and self-love. The only issue was, it was a dysfunctional strategy, and it caused major nervous system dysregulation and eventually body system burnout.

When I realised that I was not broken, I worked perfectly, and that I created my current results from an act of self-protection, my life changed. After getting over the initial shock, I realised that if I had created my body burnout, I could then recreate something new. I had the power to create a new reality.

And you do too!

Here are some reflective questions to get started on becoming aware of where you're at right now, so you can take ownership of your present state and take back your power:

- What symptoms/health issues do you have that you don't want?
- How are these health issues impacting your life? What are they costing in your relationships, your finances, your business/career, your happiness? What would be the worst case scenario, if you didn't address your body burnout? Could it lead to a divorce? To psychologically messing up your kids? To losing your business or quitting your job? To not being able to pay the mortgage? To living a sick and soul-less life forever, never ever tapping into your true potential?
- What unhealthy behaviours or thought patterns are derailing you?
- What do you honestly believe about yourself? When you get brutally honest, do you believe you are enough? Or are you inadequate, bad, broken, unworthy, unlovable, insecure, dangerous?

- How could your state of health actually be working for you? What dysfunctional patterns of behaviour can you notice that are actually serving or protecting you? What needs are being met?
- Is it possible for you to believe that you are actually not a victim, but the creator of your current health state?
- Are you ready to take 100% responsibility of your health and your life?

Where do I want to go?

Now that you are aware of your present state, you are ready to create a new dream for yourself. It's time to get super clear on where you want to go. Some questions to get you started:

- Who do you want to be? What does that mum/partner/boss/career woman/friend look like?
- How does your body feel? What does it look like?
- What can you do with your recharged body?
- How do you emotionally and spiritually feel?
- What new behavioural habits have you adopted, to become who you want to be?
- What new empowering beliefs do you have about yourself, to become this new version of yourself?
- What does your life now look like?
- WHY do you want these things? What do these things give you?
- What are the costs of getting these things? Do the benefits outweigh the costs?

You want to clearly see your new self. You want to be able to taste it. You want to be able to feel it, viscerally in your soul. This will create a strong desire, an unstoppable motivation to *become* this new woman. Getting super clear on *why* your new vision of yourself is important to you, is also crucial. If getting healthy doesn't feel that important to you, then it's likely that you will quit at some stage, especially when things get too hard, or too confusing, or when you're not seeing results fast enough. Your new vision of yourself needs to be so important, that it kills off any other possibilities of being. And finally, you need to understand the costs of getting what you want. What might you need to give up in order to be the healthy, vibrant woman you want to be? Are there people or lifestyle choices or thought-processes that you're going to have to cut-loose? Are you ready to give up the victim-card - blaming and excusing your current state on others or other things - and take full responsibility so you can get what you want? Most people don't go wholeheartedly after their dreams because they've never done a cost-benefit assessment. They get scared or blocked because, deep-down, subconsciously, they're actually not sure if it's worth it, or even safe to succeed.

How did I get here?

Next step: how did you wind up to where you are now, in a state of body burnout? Looking back into the past is an essential part of getting to the root-cause of why your body systems burned-out in the first place, and an essential step to moving towards your new dream of yourself. Yes, you need to consider what your diet has been like, your lifestyle, toxin exposures, past stressors, pathogenic infections, family history of diseases and genetic presuppositions, antibiotic-use, pregnancies, injuries, etc. All of these things are very important to consider, and most are covered in the other chapters. But these are all what I call "surface-level" root-causes. What many people miss when they are trying to heal from chronic illness is looking at what set the system up to be susceptible to body burnout in the first place. And this is where we come back to the deepest root-cause of dysfunctional beliefs, and uncover where they actually came from.

A child's belief-system about themselves and their existence in the world is created before the age of seven (the imprint period, as known in psychology), and that this belief-system then dictates behaviour throughout life. Some adults never review their old belief-system, and continue living-out old patterns created as a child right up until they die. The thing is, most kids will create negative meanings about themselves when they experience an event that creates an emotionally-charged negative emotion, like humiliation, embarrassment, shame or rejection. This is the place where dysfunctional beliefs start. Going back to the past to review and deconstruct old beliefs is essential, so that you can then rewire old beliefs into more empowering ones that allow you to flourish and give you health.

When I was doing this work, there were a few key memories that kept floating to my conscious mind as I journaled and reflected. All of these memories pointed to my feelings - my child's belief - of being weak and incapable. One of these memories was of an event that caused intense embarrassment. According to David Hawkin's Map of Consciousness, humiliation is the lowest energetic emotion we can have, and is often where unkind agreements about yourself stem from.

I was about seven or so years old. I was preparing for a children's presentation at church, where all the children sat on the stage and sang songs and read talks to the audience. I had a little one minute talk written out, and I decided I was going to memorise mine and recite it on the stage without reading it. Oh how proud my mum and dad would be! I recited it perfectly at home. I was so pleased with myself. But, then…the day of the presentation. I got up on the stage and my mind went completely and utterly blank. I turned beet red and burst out crying and ran back to my seat on the stage! The worse part: I had to sit on the stage completely humiliated and ashamed, with 100 people from the audience looking at me, while all the other little kids got up and spoke their talks perfectly. Why could they all do their talks, without freaking out and crying? My childish conclusion was that there must've been something wrong with me, that I must've been inherently weak and incapable.

As time unfolded, other events validated this misdirected belief, carving it deeper into my unconscious state and into every cell of my body. This set up patterns of anxiousness, shyness and a fear of speaking out loud. And later lead to perfectionism and obsessively studying at school to get good grades as a teen in an attempt to prove I was smart, and to hide from being found out that I was weak and incapable. My nervous system became super dysregulated, and even as a teen I started having hormonal issues and vasovagal episodes where I would faint, fit and pee myself when my body was under even a little extra stress (like pulling off a bandaid!). Over-doing, high-achieving and never feeling like I could "relax" continued into my adult years, leading to further nervous system dysregulation and body system burnout. Having kids was the last straw that broke the camel's back!

Identifying where my beliefs stemmed from, and being able to name the dysfunctional belief with exactness (i.e. weak and incapable) was essential to then be able to review, deconstruct and reframe it. I went back as an adult with more awareness, capacity and empathy, to see what else could've been true in that moment. What other stories could I have created? Well, firstly, no other kid even tried to memorise their talk - so kudos to me for being brave and strong enough for trying. And secondly, I was vulnerable enough to cry in front of 100 people, which is a sign of strength (able to express emotions) not weakness. As an adult, I was able to go back and give the child a kinder way of seeing herself, and provide her with a more empowering belief: you are strong and capable, you always have been. You were born pure potential, you are of divine worth. You are light and you are love! This allowed me to enter a more empowered state, to create new neural pathways with my new belief, without it feeling empty or forced (or unsafe!), which is often the case when you're just trying to recite positive affirmations without having done the awareness and review work of what your dysfunctional belief is, where it came from, and why it's there (to protect you).

How will I get there?

Ok, so now you know where your belief-system started, which lead to your burnout in the first place, now it's time to become the healthy, vibrant, successful woman you want to be. Yes there will be physical healing to do, to really get your body systems functioning optimally. And yes you'll need to clean up your environment to make it conducive to healing. I'll tap into these later in the book. But in order to make all this possible, healing must start from within. It starts by reprogramming new, more empowering beliefs about yourself, your body, and your ability to be whole and well.

Once you've uncovered your deep fear - the dysfunctional belief you have about yourself - now it's time to flip it. For me, for example, I flipped my old belief that I was weak and incapable, to being strong and capable. Don't get me wrong, this didn't happen overnight. Decades of believing I was defected meant I had created pretty strong neural pathways - every cell in my body was responding to this, and it was showing up in my thoughts, feelings, behaviours, health and in life. I had to work really intentionally towards reprogramming my brain and create new neural pathways. But the beautiful thing is: we can change "entrenched" beliefs, thought and behavioural patterns. Neuroscience backs this up. Scientists show that it takes an average of 66 days for old neural pathways to disintegrate, as new ones are created in place. What you repetitively say to yourself, what you think, how you act, will all impact the way you are wired. Here are some powerful techniques to reprogram deep-seated beliefs:

Inner Dialogue
Louise Hay, in her book, *Heal Your Body*, claims that all ailments are due to mental causes. For example, a probable mental cause of constipation could be a refusal to release old ideas, or being stuck in the past. Hay says health issues can be overcome with new thought patterns (and she has a great deal of experience, after curing herself from cancer using the power of the mind).

Embodied Declarations
Positive affirmations can be powerful reprogramming tools - if done in a way that guides the unconscious mind to change beliefs. Most people parrot affirmations like "I am good enough" in the mirror using the conscious mind. If your unconscious believes you aren't good enough, what part of your mind is going to win? The unconscious mind, of course, because it makes up 95% of the mind. It will be like: "yeah, whatever, we don't believe

that!" Judith Richards, creator of The Richards Trauma Process (TRTP), a modality I use in our practice, cracked the code for reprogramming unconscious core beliefs. She taught me that throwing your body into the process, viscerally *feeling* your new declarations, and saying them with conviction will cut past the conscious mind. Also using the words "I choose to know it's safe for me…" will also guide the unconscious to choose to know something new - and that it's safe to do so.

Richly Imagine
The language of the unconscious is the imagination. When you can richly imagine a new reality for yourself - consistently, everyday - you will start naturally moving towards this. This is because the unconscious doesn't know the difference between what you experience in reality and what you richly imagine. When your unconscious mind is onboard with this new you, your thought patterns, behavioural patterns and even your physical symptoms will naturally start changing.

Switch-Off Trauma
Often dysfunctional beliefs are tied up with traumatic or distressing events. Instead of these events being stored in the hippocampus as memory, trauma gets stuck in the unconscious, going round and round like broken video-tape loops, as if they are happening now, keeping you in a hyper-vigilant state. In order to detach these beliefs, often distressing events need to be addressed as well with unconscious change-work. For some of our clients, trauma has been resolved in as little as 2-weeks.

Daily Awareness
There will be unconscious resistance when you are doing reprogramming work. So while it's important to plug in specific time to dedicate yourself to practices, even more important is to stay aware of any old beliefs or dysfunctional patterns that pop up as you live your life. When you are "triggered," take a step back and thank the old belief/pattern for protecting you for so long. But then tell the old belief/ pattern that you're choosing to try a different way of thinking and being now, and that it's safe to do so.

The cool thing is, you can use similar unconscious practices to also change the way your body has coded and is experiencing symptoms - with practice and consistency, you can learn to literally turn off symptoms.

What is going to stop me?
You've got your action plan, a guide to help you, and you're leaning into the process with your own innate healing power. Many people enter the healing journey thinking healing will happen in a perfect upward line from point A to point B. Unfortunately, it never happens that way. It's more like a curly, up and down, tangled line that eventually (with consistency, effort and addressing issues from different angles) gets you to your desired result. Because of this, you need to be ready for all potential obstacles. The last step to ensure you move forward with empowerment and unstoppable motivation, is to get clear on all the ways you could get "blocked" from getting to where you want to be. They could be:

- Your current level of health might stop you from doing the things you need to do to address root-causes
- Family members might sabotage your good intentions
- Time-issues - how can I fit in self-care in my already very long list of to-do's?
- Finances, or more correctly, money mindset around what you value
- Not seeing fast enough results, and quitting too early
- Chasing the shiny unicorn, like the next best thing on Dr Google, rather than sticking to a plan
- Unaddressed self-limiting beliefs, holding you back
- Unprocessed past trauma or negative memories, keeping you stuck
- A flaky WHY - your WHY isn't strong enough to make healing the *only* possibility

This list could go on, and would be different for each person. Brainstorm your own list of obstacles that might stop you from achieving your goals, and then make a plan for how you will act, if these issues pop up along your journey (which they more than likely will at some point!).

"If, Then...Planning" is a great tool to do this. With "If, Then...Planning," you think about all the ways you could fall off track, and create a plan of attack *if* it were to happen. Rather than being reactive in the moment when things aren't "ideal," you will already have thought up all the potential obstacles that could cause you to go off track, and you've made a plan for what you would do in that moment. Reality first happens in the mind, before it happens in real life. So pre-plan your reality!

An example...*If* you have slept in and you don't have time to make a healthy lunch to take to work, you will *then* head to your local health cafe and order the cleanest (and yummiest!) looking salad. *If* the cafe happens to be closed, you will *then* head to the supermarket and purchase a pre-packaged salad and a can of tuna. *If* the supermarket has sold out of these items (unlikely!), *then* you will...and so on. You can also use "If, Then...Planning" from a mindset point of view. For example, *if* you get triggered emotionally by feeling like you have no time to look after yourself, *then* take a step back and ask yourself: "is this really a time issue, or an opinion issue? Am I going back to the old story of not being capable of healing (for example), and just using time as the excuse?"

Scan for book resources

You can download a copy of our "**If, Then...Planning**" at - www.chrisandfilly.fm/book

Now that you're in an empowered state, and have unlocked your healing potential, let's take a deeper look into the nervous system, and the importance of achieving a calm mind, even in the face of stress.

SUMMARY
EXPOWERED MIND

As a summary, here's what you need to do to become empowered, to rewire your brain and your beliefs, so that you can heal:

- Understand and acknowledge that self-limiting beliefs are almost always at the core of body burnout.
- Get painfully clear on where you're at now and what body burnout is costing you, so that the current cost is greater than the cost of change.
- Create a powerful dream and strong why about who you want to be, so compelling that it creates healing and ending your body burnout as the *only* option.
- Understand how you got to this point of body burnout, and the deepest root-causes - your dysfunctional beliefs, and where they all began.
- Get to work creating new beliefs, and retraining your brain to heal your thoughts, feelings, behaviours and body.
- Brainstorm all the obstacles that could get in the way of becoming who you want to be, and create a plan on how you will address them, when they pop up.

CHAPTER 5

Calm Mind

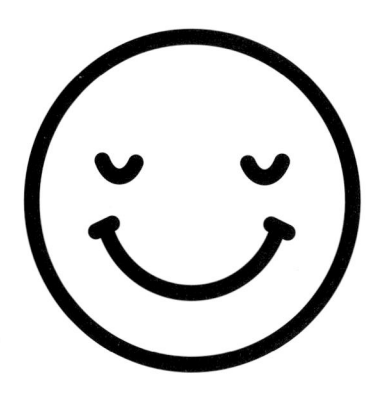

Introduction

Let's talk about stress, baby! The whole purpose of getting into an empowered state by reprogramming unhealthy beliefs and stories, is to not only change thought and behavioural patterns that lead to burnout, but, even more importantly, to create a calm mind and internal resistance, especially in the face of stress. Because, let's face it, stress is always going to be part of your life. But it's how you *respond* to stress, that will be the real winner in your healing and optimal health journey.

Stress is the number one cause of chronic illness. In fact, data reports that 75-90% of all physician office visits are for stress-related ailments, especially due to work-life-family imbalances. Stress not only leads to body burnout and energy, mood and gut issues, but it has also been linked to the six leading causes of death: heart disease, cancer, lung ailments, accidents, cirrhosis of the liver and suicide. I don't think I need to say much else for you to agree that stress is a killer, and that learning to calm your farm is absolutely essential. Am I right? Say "yes!" with me sister!

In this chapter, I dive deeper into how stress affects your nervous system, the many facets of stress, how pain acts as a signal to keep us safe, and how you can become a healthy stress-responding queen.

Nervous system 101

Ok, let's talk first about the nervous system - the system that controls your stress-response. Your nervous system is your body's command centre, involving your brain, spinal cord and a complex network of nerves to all areas of your body. It is responsible for receiving and processing sensory information, and for controlling the body's responses to that information. It is constantly sending messages back and forth between the brain and the body, based on the external environment, what is happening in your body, and how you're interpreting all this based on your belief-systems stored in your unconscious mind. The nervous system is hardwired to keep us alive. It controls the function of all other body systems. And it is also constantly scanning the external environment, and responding to any physical or mental-emotional (metaphysical) "threats."

When you're feeling safe, relaxed, and at ease, you switch into the parasympathetic nervous system response, which allows you to rest, digest, and assists healthy functioning of all other body systems. When you feel "threatened" your nervous system jumps into survival mode, and switches into the sympathetic nervous system state, the "stressed-state," which alerts your body to either fight, flee or freeze from the impending danger. It's natural and normal to switch in and out of the parasympathetic and sympathetic nervous systems, however, when you're chronically stuck in the sympathetic state, your nervous system becomes super dysregulated, which has a damaging impact on all other body systems. In this state, your neuroendocrine system chronically fires off cortisol and adrenaline, leading to adrenal fatigue, neurotransmitter depletion and suppression of sex hormones. Your gut will also switch off, because you're not able to digest food effectively in the sympathetic nervous system state. Your immune system will suppress, leading to pathogenic infections and autoimmunity. And your detoxification system will also malfunction, as blood flow leaves your internal organs, to give more energy to your external limbs (legs and arms) so you can "fight" or "flee."

> **Scan for book resources**
>
> To get an understanding of the health of your nervous system, head to www.chrisandfilly.fm/book for an instructional on how to assess your nervous system by looking at your vagus nerve (the nerve that connects your brain to your body's organs) using a simple at-home self-test, as well as easy vagus nerve toning exercises you can do at home.

So, in essence, your body systems burnout when your nervous system becomes dysregulated. I've identified the two main sources of "stress" that dysregulate the nervous system - physical inflammation and metaphysical inflammation (as shown in figure 5.1).

Physical inflammation includes things like environmental toxins, processed foods, parasites, genetic mutations, etc. I'll go into more of these in a sec. But for now, all you need to know is that physical sources of inflammation will put the nervous system into a state of stress, because they can pose real physiological dangers to the body. Chronic exposure, then, will lead to nervous system dysregulation and body system breakdown. However, there are some people out there eating takeaway, living in a

Figure 5.1: Cause of Body Burnout

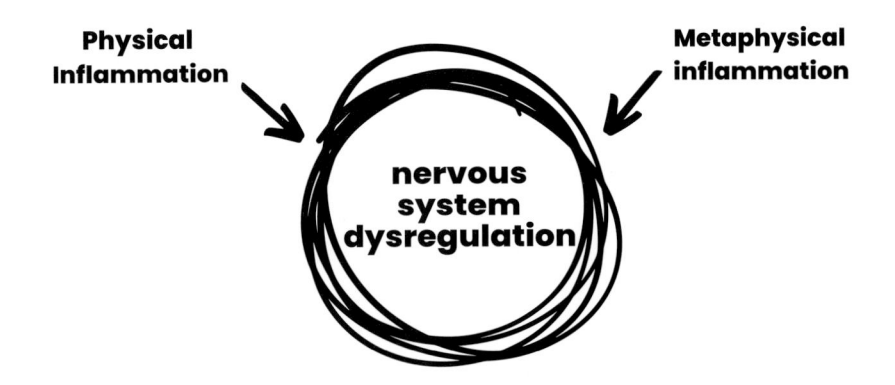

Physical Inflammation → nervous system dysregulation ← **Metaphysical inflammation**

mouldy environment, and with genetic mutations, yet they are cruising through life just fine. (Yep, I'm hearing you, thinking how unfair that is when you try so hard to get well, yet you're still stuck in a state of body burnout!). So what's the difference here? Why can some people be exposed to physical inflammatory triggers and cruise along fine, while other people don't? It often comes back to the deepest root-cause of burnout: dysfunctional beliefs, which can cause "metaphysical inflammation."

Dysfunctional beliefs are major contributors of nervous system dysregulation, because you're living with your beliefs of shame, guilt, unworthiness, fear, etc., 24/7, and they're very often hidden in your unconscious state and trapped in the cells of your body, as clinically researched in Dr Nicole LePera's (aka The Holistic Psychologist) book *How To Do The Work*. These beliefs, as I touched upon in the previous chapter, wire your nervous system into a state of stress. You're constantly needing to prove, defend, hide or run away. Your nervous system responds to internal emotional-mental stress in just the same way as it would from a physical stressor. Both will release cortisol and adrenaline, and switch off your gut and detox pathways. This is why we call dysfunctional beliefs and mental-emotional imbalances "metaphysical inflammation," because, just like alcohol or toxic chemicals, they are physically inflammatory! In his book, *Gut Feelings*, functional medicine expert Dr Will Cole calls the stress, shame and trauma that inflames the gut and other body systems "Shameflammation."

In addition, dysfunctional beliefs create an abnormal stress response towards your day-to-day stressors - be that finances, the ratty kids, work demands, health issues - because you're constantly on-guard, feeling threatened, unsafe and insecure. How can you manage in any area of your life, if deep down, unconsciously, you believe there is something wrong with you?

The more chaotic your conscious and unconscious mind become, the more you can produce inflammation in your body, and become more susceptible to external physical inflammatory sources. And the more inflamed your body becomes, the more it can cause further chaos in your mind. It can become a sticky, vicious cycle! As Dr Will Cole rightly says: "mental health IS physical health." Amen Dr Cole. The body and mind are deeply and intricately connected.

Breaking down stressors

Ok, so let's breakdown the different types of stressors, so you can clearly see what you're dealing with when it comes to ending your body burnout. Holistic health expert, Paul Chek identified 6 main stressors that affect the *whole* self. The first five stressors fall under "physical inflammation." I'll tap into these physical stressors in more detail later in this book. For now, here's a quick summary below:

Physical

Body system burnout is the biggest physical stressor: hormonal imbalances, gut inflammation, detox issues, neurotransmitter depletion and chronic muscular-skeletal injuries and pain. Women who are mums also have the extra physical stressor of pregnancy, birth, breastfeeding and sleepless nights. Even if you had a lovely pregnancy and birth, and breastfeeding is a breeze, your little munchkin will be sucking all the nutrients from you, which is literally "stressing" to your system. And for some mid-life mums, their bodies don't bounce back, even years after child-bearing. And exercise! While it's great and healthy, over-exercising will burn your body out.

Chemical
Chemical stressors include environmental toxins, like petrol fumes, paints, solvents, factory gasses, sprays, as well as toxic mould. Nasty chemicals in your skincare and cleaning products can also add to your stress bucket. Then you can have natural chemicals in foods, like histamine, salicylates and sulphur, which can cause stress and inflammation in susceptible people with chemical sensitivities.

Electromagnetic
Electromagnetic fields (or EMF's) can also add to your stress bucket. Unless you live out in the bush, off-grid without any reception, you are likely exposed to a ton of EMF's. These come from electrical appliances in your home, computers, laptops, mobile phones, bluetooth devices and 4G/5G. They are what I call "silent" stressors.

Nutrition
Man-made, synthetic foods are inflammatory to the body. Things like trans-fats, refined carbs and processed sugars. Poor quality "healthy" food can also add to your stress load - things like grain-fed, caged animal products and plants sprayed with Roundup. Skipping meals unintentionally, eating on the run, and eating reactive (even healthy) foods are also stressful.

Thermal
Thermal stress is pretty simple. You're either too hot or you're too cold. This could be due to environmental issues, like not having sufficient heating or airflow in your home. It could also be a result of hormonal imbalances that can affect your internal temperature.

Psychic
The last type of stress - psychic stress - falls under the mental-emotional "metaphysical inflammation" sources of stress. It's all the stuff that keeps your brain wired and feeling overwhelmed - kids, work, deadlines, to-do's, relationship issues, finances, self-doubt, guilt, shame, fear. Bottling up how you feel and repressing

trauma (no matter how big or small) is also a form of psychic stress that can cause body burnout symptoms. Unprocessed emotions get stored as energy in the body, and if not released, the unprocessed emotion will instead try to surface physically in the body through pain, as clinically demonstrated in Bessell Van der Kolk's book *The Body Keeps The Score*. Studies also show emotional suppression has been linked to chronic diseases, including cancer.

At the crux of psychic stress is how you think and feel about yourself, and the beliefs and stories you have created about yourself, which dictate how you behave and respond to emotional stressors. I hope I've harped on about this enough already, for you to understand that this is always at the deepest root-cause of body burnout.

As you can see, stress isn't just about the bills stacking up. There are so many ways your body and mind can become overwhelmed, which inevitably lead to nervous system dysregulation and your body systems crumbling. The more stressors filling your bucket, the greater the likelihood of symptoms arising - and if it goes on long enough unchecked, premature death! You definitely don't want that happening, now, do you beautiful lady?

Scan for book resources

Many people get stuck even knowing where to start with dealing with all potential stressors. This is often because people try to control what's outside of their control, or they feel helpless in trying to control anything. Clearly identifying your own unique stressors, and identifying what you have control over, can help you step out of overwhelm and into a space of empowerment and calm.

Head to www.chrisandfilly.fm/book to download our "**Identifying & Addressing Stressors**" guide, which helps you break your stressors down into bite-sized chunks so you can create a step-by-step action-plan to move out of overwhelm.

Pain as a loving message

When stressors fill up your bucket too much, physical pain is the inevitable outcome.

I used to hate pain. And don't get me wrong, I'll still get frustrated when it shows up. But what I've come to learn is that pain is simply a signal that something is out of balance. Going back to the nervous system - pain is designed to keep us safe, to grab our attention that something needs to be addressed. This pain mechanism is how humans evolved and survived.

Pain will, at some point, arise when there is physical inflammation and body system imbalances. Most people are aware that a health symptom - bloating, acne, headaches, painful periods - is a message from the body that something physical is out of balance. If you're someone who pushes through pain, your first step is to practice listening, more intently, more lovingly, to the pain in your body. What is it trying to tell you? Where is the pain coming from? What body system might need supporting? What inflammatory trigger might need to be extinguished? Pain does not exist to hurt or annoy you. Pain is not a sign that your body is fighting *against* you. It's actually a sign that your body is fighting *for* you - it's a hard-wired mechanism created to grab your attention to motivate you to find homeostasis again. If you're reading this book, it's highly likely pain has grabbed your attention and motivated you to start looking for answers about your body burnout. This act alone shows us that pain is actually a loving message, leading us back to safety and alignment. Without pain, there can be no healing (only eventual and sudden death). So next time you have a flare up of pain, place your hand on the source of pain, and thank it for the message it is trying to send you, and get to work identifying the source.

Now, let's go a level deeper. Yes, there must be a physiological response or imbalance causing the pain, but the root of that pain often lies in the unconscious state. When you are out of alignment with your self, when you're feeding into dysfunctional beliefs and stories about yourself, every cell in your body also feels unsafe. The unconscious mind can't verbally talk to us, so it uses physical pain to grab our attention.

Let me explain this with my heartburn story. I mentioned earlier that my health issues flared up again in 2020 when the COVID-19 pandemic hit. One symptom that was really incessant was heartburn. I healed the heartburn physically with gut-protocols a few years earlier, when my health initially crumbled after having kids. So I thought: *it's all good, I've got this, I'll just do the same protocols and the heartburn will clear up*. This time, however, all the physical protocols didn't budge the heartburn. I quickly learned that I couldn't out-supp or out-diet the deepest root-cause - the physical healing only "stuck" for a few years. I needed to dig deeper.

This is when I came across a passage in Jaemin Frazer's book, *Unhindered*: "Your body craves health. Health is the default. When you take the handbrake off and give yourself permission to flourish, health is where you end up. Being unhealthy, sick and carrying excess weight is serving you by protecting you from what you are most afraid of."

The thing I was most afraid of was the fear of being weak and incapable. It made sense that the heartburn flared up during COVID when there was heightened "stress" and so many things out of my control. My unconscious state turned on the pain - the heartburn (physically, by increasing stress hormones, shutting off digestive juices, and releasing histamines) - to grab my attention. And it wasn't letting me off the hook this time with relief using supps or diets. This time, it was going to ensure I got to the bottom of things!

And so I did. It took four and a half months of doing deep inner healing, reprogramming new beliefs, rewiring the brain and regulating the nervous system, for the heartburn to lift. I remember the day that it happened. I had been experiencing heartburn pretty much daily, and after a coaching session with my coach, where I'd experienced some really cool emotional shifts, I ate dinner that night. It was a meal high in histamine - tomatoes, spices, GF pasta - a meal I'd eaten for lunch and dinner the previous two days earlier, that had "given" me heartburn. But this time, after I ate, I spoke to my body.

You've got this body. I trust you. I love you. You're whole. You're well. You're fighting for me, not against me. I believe in you. I believe in me. I am strong. I am capable. I am amazing. Body you are amazing. And I'm so sorry. I'm so truly sorry I had been doubting you, when I didn't even consciously know I had been!

And as I spoke to my body. The most beautiful thing happened. From the top of my throat right to the bottom of my gut, I felt the most intense rippling feelings of energy and light and love cascade from one end of my gut to the other. I can't explain it in any other way then I was spiritually being healed.

With my empty bowl of food in front of me, I burst out crying. Tears of awe. Tears of gratitude. Tears of forgiveness. Tears of pure love for my self and my amazing body. And there was no heartburn. NO heartburn! Even when logically, this meal, this starchy, high-histaminey meal, *should've* triggered the heartburn! And for two days after that, every time I ate, I felt the same spiritual, energetic, rippling feelings of love and light from my throat to the bottom of my gut - and no heartburn!

I've been heartburn-free since - *except* when I had broken rapport with myself, or had fallen out of alignment with myself. Like when I started agreeing with old dysfunctional beliefs about myself, or when I started running old dysfunctional patterns, like addictive-doing or feeling like I needed to prove or defend. When this had occurred, the heartburn switched on, a loving message from my unconscious state, telling me very clearly that I had gone out of alignment. And as soon as I realigned with myself, the heartburn switched off - *immediately*!

How freaking amazing are our bodies, that we can communicate with our unconscious state, via our nervous system, through pain? We have everything inside of us to heal, to be whole, to be calm, and to be happy.

When I've shared this heartburn story with others, many have said: "Wow, you're so in tune with your body. I wish I was that in tune." Am I special to have had this deep healing experience? No, not at all! Anyone, when willing, can learn to communicate with their body. In fact, it's how we're hardwired - you just have to learn how to get out of your own way. This, my friend, is the key to ending your body burnout and becoming intimately in tune with your self, your body and finding inner peace and calm (regardless of what's going on around you).

SUMMARY
CALM MIND

❺

As a summary, here's what you need to do to master a calm mind:

- Understand how the nervous system works, and the interconnection between your brain, nerves, body, conscious and unconscious mind.
- Get clear on all the different types of stressors, and identify and address stressors you have control over.
- Learn to listen to the messages your body is sending you, and work with your pain, not against it, to restore homeostasis and realign with yourself.
- Now it's time to get practical - to get organised - so you can do the things you need to do to end your body burnout, and become the type of woman you truly desire!

CHAPTER 6

Organised Mind

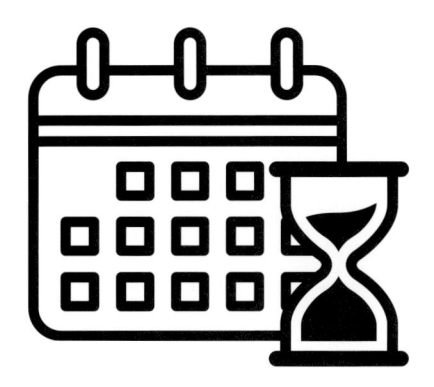

Introduction

If you've tapped into your own internal power, reprogrammed self-limiting beliefs, have a steadfast and compelling *why,* and have learned to listen to the messages from your body and your unconscious state, tapping into your own inner calm, the rest of the things in this book will come naturally, actioned by a deep love and honour for yourself.

In this chapter, we get practical. I breakdown a very handy process, that will help you become super organised, so you can take action and implement the things you need to do to address root-causes, and heal from body burnout.

Too often, busy, high-achieving women burnout because they are torn between a million different things - work, kids, partner, self-care, hobbies, friends, cleaning, cooking - and constantly feeling frazzled and overwhelmed. Am I right? When you get to this point, you struggle to think straight, and you likely burn energy you don't have (your *future* energy!), wire-up your nervous system, and get stuck doing things that don't matter, or that don't get you anywhere. The more you do, blindly, in a high cortisol/adrenaline state, the more you burn your body systems out. A disorganised, chaotic mind and lifestyle absolutely affect your health, and your ability to implement a treatment plan and heal yourself. In the words of Benjamin Franklin: "By failing to prepare, you're preparing to fail."

After reading this chapter, you will see why mastering an organised mind is key to healing. You will also have practical steps to take, to help you become an organisational queen, aligning your health, happiness and your vision for yourself, with your priorities - with flow, rather than forcing the outcome.

Last on your "to-do" list - Rose's story

Rose was juggling many balls. Kids, business, cooking, cleaning, farm work, admin, volunteering at the kids school, family activities, taxi-ing, paying the bills. As you saw earlier, Rose was stuck in motherhood martyrdom, doing everything for everyone else, and leaving herself last.

Through coaching around self-limiting beliefs, Rose became "aware" of her motherhood martyrdom patterns. She got it. She understood it. She saw where it came from. She acknowledged it was at the deepest root-cause of her body burnout. Yet she struggled, initially, to change her behavioural patterns.

"I can see where my health issues are stemming from, but I'm really struggling to do the things I need to do to heal. Even taking my supplements - I know I *feel better* when I take them, but I keep forgetting to take the doses."

We dug into the blocks stopping her from putting her health first. First up, Rose had only stopped at "awareness" of her dysfunctional belief of being unlovable and how that was feeding into her motherhood martyrdom patterns. She was struggling to "find time" to reprogram her beliefs and retrain her brain, which meant anything else she needed to do was going to be tossed out the window. In order to lean into the process, and start seeing a transformation that would naturally lead to honouring herself, Rose needed help with getting her life organised, so she could carve out time to do her healing program.

Currently, from the moment Rose woke, to when she fell asleep, she dove into doing-doing-doing for others. She woke when the kids woke, got them dressed, fed, lunchboxes done, drove them to school. Returned home and started treating clients, back to back, with little time in between. When the kids came home, she did the housework, made dinner, put the kids to bed, then crashed to bed herself in a state of exhaustion (that's if her husband wasn't pining for sex!). Rose had major scheduling issues that were not only exhausting her, but that were also affecting her ability to do her inner work, feed herself nourishing food, take her lab-based healing supplements, recover and fill up her energy stores, and find joy in her day-to-day life.

Until Rose could create a new schedule that would give space to prioritising herself first, she would continue to flounder, only implementing her healing program 25%, and only seeing 25% of the results, if that.

Stay tuned for the organisational process that helped Rose gain momentum.

Over-valuing work - Hazel's story

Hazel, as you have learned, was obsessed with working. Obsessed to the point where it was literally burning out her body systems. She'd work at 110%, kicking goals, working up the corporate ladder. She'd bring work home, and continue to work after the kids went to bed. Her health, and even her relationship with her two boys, were put on the back-burner. In the end, her body was screaming at her to stop - literally screaming pain from her gut. To give her the message she needed, her health issues put a brake on what she valued highly - work, and her productivity to work.

You discovered earlier, that Hazel's deepest root-cause came from her feeling of inadequacy and needing to "prove" herself. This inner reprogramming was hard for Hazel to change. To face up to her deepest fears of inadequacy, meant that she would have to relinquish her obsession with work, and organise her life in a new way, that would give space for healing her body, her heart, and connect with her children.

But what Hazel found, as she leaned into her root-causes, was that she could carve space for health, family, and still be productive at work. By doing less "work," she was actually able to achieve more, because she had greater physical and mental-emotional capacity.

I'll share very soon, the resources Hazel used, to organise her life with healthy balance.

A disorganised mess - Isla's story

Isla's anxiety made her mind feel like a disorganised mess. On the outside, she fluttered around like a butterfly. Beautiful and colourful and outgoing. A vibrant hair salon business owner and boss. The life of the party. But inside she was crippled with anxiety, chaos, messiness, and this showed up in how she lived her life. She had no structure, no routines. She winged it in her business. Her relationship with her partner was an emotional rollercoaster. And her health was a yo-yo - swinging from eating strict Keto, to bingeing out on all the food and wine, then excessively gyming to burn off the "shameful" calories. When her anxiety ramped up, these patterns only got worse. Her life felt like a disorganised mess.

As you discovered, Isla's deepest root-cause was steeped in childhood trauma, and the stories she created around the sexual abuse to make sense of what had happened. And that was: she was unworthy, she was not enough. Isla made some headway with addressing her self-limiting beliefs, and while this took the edge off her anxiety, she was still struggling to create healthier behaviours.

"I feel like the state of my body is stopping me from moving forward."

Isla was a case where her physiology was closely linked to her psychology. She needed a two-pronged approach. As she prioritised taking her therapeutic lab-based supplements to restore her serotonin levels and rebalance her hormones, the anxiety improved, which gave her further inner calm to continue working on her self-limiting beliefs, and structure a more healthy, and consistent lifestyle.

Bringing your dream into reality

In Chapter 4, you created a strong dream for your future self. You clearly saw, felt, even tasted, who you wanted to be, and what that felt and looked like. Becoming a visionary allows you to step out of victim mode, and take full responsibility for where you're at now, and where you're going. But what's even more powerful, is creating that dream. In the next sections, I take you through, step-by-step, how you can turn your dream into reality.

Lovely, it's time to become your own creator. It's time to put your dream into action!

Goals

Stephen Covey famously said: "All things are created twice - first in your mind, then in reality." Goals are the stepping stones that make your vision a reality. They should be SMART - specific, measurable, achievable, relevant and time-bound. The problem with goals is that many people set goals that have no connection to their vision. Think about all the New Years Resolutions you have made. Lose 10kgs. Swim in the ocean daily. Quit sugar. Double your revenue. Be more positive. Most goals are virtuous, and are often made to better yourself - or your circumstances. But did you create them based on your new dream of yourself? Did you even have a vision of who you wanted to be? Most people don't. Most goals are plucked from the air because they sound good, or because you feel like you *should* be doing that thing. Whenever the word "should" or "need to" comes into your vocabulary, be very wary. No one ever achieves anything because they feel like they "should" or "need to."

Plucking goals out of thin air, that don't align with your vision, will only end in failure. Your unconscious mind knows when you've made a goal that doesn't align with what you deeply want. And it will constantly sabotage you from achieving that goal.

Projects

In order to make your goals achievable, you need to break them down into chunks, or what we call projects. Projects are things that you do, make, get or become. They are things that can be ticked off, and which lead you to achieving your goal, and ultimately your dream of yourself.

Not breaking down goals into manageable chunks, is where many people go wrong when they try to heal their body. There are often many things you need to do, become and implement in order to heal body systems. Very often people become overwhelmed, and scramble around trying to get well, flitting from one thing to the next, without a system, process or focus. No wonder so many people give up trying to get healthy!

Tasks

To achieve your projects, you have to break the project down into even smaller tasks. Tasks often look like your to-do's. Things that need to be ticked off, in order to achieve your project. I'm a big believer of taking "small steps." Making small changes, implementing small things over time, is not only achievable (especially if you're in a state of overwhelm!), but also sustainable. Chris's motto when he coaches our clients is: 1% better each day. Totally achievable, right?

Habits

Now you can have some tasks that you do once, or for a short period, and you're done. However, many tasks are often repeatable, that you do over and over again, most likely daily. These are essential things like drinking water, eating and sleeping. Or things that you want to incorporate into your daily life, like restorative movement, inner work, or being present with your family. Some habits can be done on top of each other, at the same time. Like going for a walk with your family (restorative movement, plus being present with your family). These repeatable tasks make up your habits, which make up your lifestyle, and who you are. In order to truly embody these new habits, you will need to practice them regularly, and live them as if you already are the type of person who has these habits. Using a habit tracker to keep yourself accountable and to measure your progress is super helpful. But you'll also intuitively know when you've mastered new habits by who you are and how you feel.

Tools

Using tools - the last step in our organisational process - will help you to save so much time and mental space. Tools could look like using a whiteboard and sticky notes, a dedicated notebook, a card deck, an app, or a combination of all three. Whatever tool you choose, it should include space to track your vision, goals, projects, tasks and habits, as well as your daily living schedule so you can time-block when you will action tasks, as well as take into account activities happening that week for yourself, family and business/work. Having everything in place will save you time, sanity, and it will make it a heck of a lot easier to actually put your vision into action.

Now, you might be reading all this and thinking: *Filly, when am I even going to have time to plan all this? I'm already feeling stretched!*

You know what? I felt exactly the same. Chris has always been the "Organised King" in our team, fully embracing this process. This was actually a huge weakness for him, something that was really holding him back from overcoming his own body burnout. He had to do a ton of personal development and implementation around getting organised, so he could prioritise the important things. In fact, the process I have outlined above was created by Chris, after trialling many different organisational methods.

When Chris presented me with this process, initially I had the same objections. I'm a "get stuff done" type of woman, and my "to-do" list was pretty much up in my head. I thought: *if I have to take timeout to write out my goals and projects and tasks and track my habits, it's going to take away my precious time to actually do the things!*

The thing is, I had so much going on inside my head, that my whole nervous system was taxed. And while I was very good at getting stuff done, and even doing the "healthy things," I was doing it out of force and fear (which stemmed from my own dysfunctional belief of being weak and incapable to manage my life). Getting out of my head and connecting to my heart and my dream of myself, helped me to align my "to-do" list with the most important stuff. I was able to clearly see all the unimportant "stuff" I was doing and let go of that stuff, and focus my attention and energy on specific goals that grounded me into my pure potential, and that led me closer to my evolved self. The whole process was extremely empowering.

There's a quote that I love from Eleanor Roosevelt: "It's takes as much time to wish, as it does to plan." It really does! And the downer is that wishing will get you nowhere, except further overwhelm, disappointment and body burnout. So, centre back into your new empowered story that you have started recreating about yourself. This will have a natural overflow of getting your life on track. Set aside some time and map out your dream of yourself and goals as a start. Then start working on one of your goals, by breaking it down into projects, tasks and habits (if appropriate). Momentum will come.

Bringing her new self to life – Hazel's story

You might be wondering what this actually looks like in real life. Let's look at how Hazel used this tool to help her get out of her addictive workaholic patterns, and align her behaviour with her dream of who she wanted to become.

Dream outcome

Hazel wanted to become:
- Healthy, vibrant, and full of energy and mental clarity
- A present, loving mum, and a good role model for her children
- Successful in her career and confident in herself – not driven to work out of force, fear and trying to prove herself

- A woman who is balanced, as well as making a big impact in the world

Goals

Hazel created goals that were stepping stones to achieving each aspect of her new self (many were interrelated). To keep it succinct, we'll map out her health goals:
- Reset adrenal stress hormones
- Clear SIBO
- Heal leaky gut and restore digestive enzymes
- Reduce inflammation

Projects

We worked on each goal, one at a time. Hazel created projects around each goal, when the time was right. For the "Clear SIBO" goal, this is what her projects looked like:
- Do the 2-week Elemental Diet (a nutritional medicine formulated shake used to clear SIBO).
- Reprogram her self-limiting belief of being inadequate, so that she could appropriately and healthily respond to stressors in her work and family life (stress was a major root-cause that was affecting her digestion and motility, which led to the SIBO in the first place).
- Bringing foods/meals back in post the Elemental Diet, safely and effectively, to prevent SIBO from flaring back up.
- Establish healthy and mindful eating patterns long-term.
- Therapeutically addressing impaired digestion and motility post the Elemental Diet, to prevent SIBO from flaring back up.

Tasks

Hazel broke each project down into tasks, so she knew exactly what she needed to do at each step, as well as how she was going to successfully implement the plan. Hazel's tasks were things that could be ticked-off after completion. Let's look at the tasks for the 2-week Elemental Diet:
- Meet with Filly to go over how to do the 2-week Elemental Diet safely and effectively.

- Purchase enough Elemental Diet formula for 2-weeks, so she doesn't run out.
- Purchase an anti-fungal (we used a fatty acid supplement, undecylenic acid) to take alongside the Elemental Diet to prevent fungal overgrowth.
- Meet with Chris to mentally prepare for the Elemental Diet, including nutting out what she will do if she begins to struggle to stay on track.
- Time-block in her schedule when she is going to start the Elemental Diet, when she is going to drink the shakes and take the anti-fungals, and when she is going to do inner work, connecting back to her new empowering self-beliefs and vision, so she could get into flow and make the process successful.

Habits

If we follow along with Hazel's Elemental Diet tasks, most of these tasks are only completed for the short-term, and didn't really need to be tracked as a new "habit." Hazel was notorious, however, for forgetting (or not prioritising?) taking her supplements, so she ended up setting reminders on her phone and tracking taking her anti-fungal pills three times a day, to help her stay on track. She also kept resisting the inner work, making the excuse that she was too busy doing "other stuff," which required more coaching around why she was holding onto old behaviours that were no longer serving her.

Now that you've elevated your mind into a more resourceful state, it's time to start implementing physical support to assist in the healing of your body.

A word of warning...

While moving towards health isn't ever a walk in the park (there will be ups and downs), it shouldn't feel like you're fighting yourself to get there. If at anytime moving towards your goals and your vision of yourself feels "forced," or like you really have to "discipline" or "manage" yourself to do the things, let this be a warning flag that you are going out of alignment with yourself.

The table below (as shown in figure 6.1), adapted from Jaemin Frazer's *Unhindered* book, is a fantastic measure of whether you are approaching your vision-making from a place of force or from flow. Flow occurs when self-permission is granted. Frazer says, self-permission can only ever come from your unconscious mind when you deeply love and trust your own nature, allowing it to be safe to show up and succeed.

I love using this table below, as a self-reflective measure to assess whether my energy of "doing" is coming from a place of self-love, kindness and trust, or if I've slipped back into old patterns of "doing" from a place of fear.

Fig 6.1 Self-Permission

SELF PERMISSION GRANTED	SELF PERMISSION NOT GRANTED
Your self-limiting beliefs have been reprogrammed. You know this because your behaviour has automatically changed, and you're seeing the results in your health and life.	Your self-limiting beliefs have not been reprogrammed. You know this because you either haven't started reprogramming, or you have started reprogramming, but not yet seeing any changes in your health or life.
You're focusing on being, which is naturally leading to doing and having the results you desire. You're focused on the "production line" not the "end product".	You're still stuck in doing and behaviour management. You're only focusing on the "end product," not the "production line," and therefore only seeing short-term gains and inconsistent results.
You're using an adult form of motivation to get what you want. As such, you are accessing the best of who you really are and what you're capable of. It feels life-giving and energy-giving.	You're still using a childish form of motivation to get what you want. You have no or little self-awareness or maturity. It is life-sucking and energy-sucking.
You are believing that you are far stronger than you ever imagined.	You're still stuck in the fear that you are weaker than you think.
You're accessing your unconscious wisdom, intuition and knowing. Your whole being is pointed in the same direction.	You're only or mostly accessing knowledge from your conscious mind, paying no or little attention to the realm of the unconscious.

You are listening, trusting, forgiving, and accepting yourself. You've released the handbrake to allow yourself to flourish and naturally move towards your goals.	You're still fighting, dominating and controlling yourself to reach your goals. It feels like you're climbing a forever snow-capped mountain, never quite reaching the top. You're violating your relationship with yourself, which can lead to further trauma.
You're listening and responding to the messages from your body, turning symptoms & pain signals off.	You're still confused and frustrated about your health issues, and don't know what your symptoms are saying to you, or how to turn them off.
You're internally validating your own worth and significance, and have become your own self-healer.	You're still externally validating your worth and significance to others, or to what you have or can do, and still outsourcing your healing to others.

SUMMARY
ORGANISED MIND

❻

As a summary, here's what you need to do to establish an organised mind, aligning your vision of your evolved self with your priorities:

- Create SMART (specific, measurable, achievable, relevant, time-bound) goals that are stepping stones to bring your new self into reality.
- When you're ready to work on a specific goal, chunk it down into smaller, achievable projects.
- From these projects, chunk it down into even smaller tasks. You may work on projects simultaneously, or one at a time.
- Identify repeatable tasks - tasks that will make up new habits. These habits should always lead to the creation of who you want to be. Track habits until they become a natural part of your being.
- Use organisational tools - whiteboard, sticky notes, notebook, apps, cards - to make this process faster, easier and effective.

STEP THREE
Heal Thy Body

STEP THREE
HEAL THY BODY

In Step Three, I go over the third step to ending your body burnout for good, and that is healing thy body. If you've done the inner mind work, this third step should be easy-peasy. Honestly: easy-peasy. You see, your body craves health. If you've gotten out of your own way by healing your mind, your behaviours will naturally move towards life-giving things. If you skipped Step Two - Heal Thy Mind because you thought you didn't need to do "mind" work, or because it was "too scary," stop right now, and go back to Step Two. Jumping straight into body work will only lead to short-term results (if any!) and frustration.

In Step Three: Heal Thy Body, I cover three essential self-care practices you need to implement to support the healing of your body systems, get your spark back, and allow yourself to shine! They are: restorative nutrition, restorative sleep and restorative movement. Good eating, sleeping and movement habits are the foundations for a healthy body. If not done right, they can absolutely contribute to burning your body systems out. On the flip side, if you are honouring your body with foods and nutrients that are supportive, if you're getting good quality, restorative sleep, and if you're moving and exercising in a way that is beneficial to your body - rather than causing *more* stress and damage - then not only can you heal your body naturally, but it will also lead to a beautiful love story of long-term health and happiness.

CHAPTER 7
Restorative Nutrition

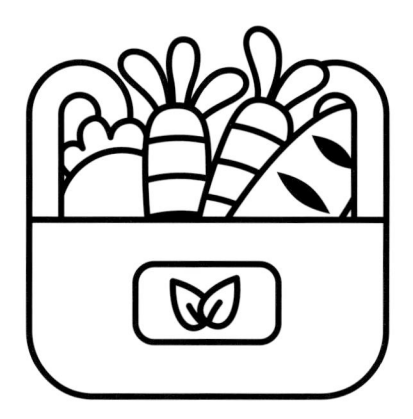

Introduction

In this chapter, you will learn all about food. Are you eating food that is poisoning your body, or is it restoring your body? Is your nutrition contributing to your body burnout? And is food enough to restore your body systems, or do you need additional therapeutical support with nutritional supplements?

Hippocrates, an ancient naturopathic doctor back in BC (I love this bloke!), famously said: "Let food be thy medicine, and medicine be thy food." Most people know, now, that food is important to health. But there are still many people who don't fully understand just how significant food is to the functioning of the body - including some medical doctors. I still have patients say to me, after seeing their medical specialist about their Irritable Bowel Disease, that their doctor brushed diet off as not being part of their disease manifestation - nor having the power to address the condition. This is mind-blowing to me, because science tells us that every cell in our body is made up of nutrients, and many of these nutrients come from the food that we eat. How could food not be part of dis-ease? And on the flip-side, surely you can support the healing of the body with the food that you eat.

After reading this chapter, you'll have a clear understanding of how to eat well for health, when you might need to use a more restrictive "healing diet," what role nutritional supplements play in healing the body systems, and how to get into flow with your eating habits.

My relationship with food

Food was where it all started for me, when I first embarked on my own healing journey. My sister gave me a book called *Deep Nutrition* by Catherine Shanahan, and it completely changed my life. The book followed the theories of Weston A. Price, which basically says we should ditch processed foods and go back to eating the way our ancestors ate - organic fruits, vegetables, meats, offal, non-pasteurised dairy, soaked and sprouted grains, nuts and seeds. It argued that our modern, "fake foods" were causing the uprise of health issues in our society - diabetes, heart disease, cancer, allergies, autoimmunity, and even dental issues due to the structural changes in our faces.

At the time of reading the book, I thought I ate "healthy" because I didn't eat McDonalds everyday. But I soon discovered my "healthy" cereal for breakfast, flimsy salad sandwiches for lunch, pasta for dinner, and sweet snacks at night, were not doing my inflamed body any favours. And so I went on a frenzy, completely transforming the way my family ate. I chucked out all the packaged, processed foods. Started making food from scratch. Shopped at the local farmer's market. My kitchen became a lab. There were legumes and spelt groats and nuts sprouting everywhere. Cabbage fermenting in jars. I even ate offal everything (until Chris started complaining that our dinners tasted like urine!). My extended family thought I was a bit nuts, and laughed at my "weird" desserts that I took to family dinners. They thought it was just a fad. But month by month, I felt the inflammation in my body calm down. And I was hooked by how good I felt.

I might've started out "dieting," but overtime this way of eating has become who I am - like quite literally, I am what I eat. I love the food that I eat. And my body loves me for it. I hope you can also develop this same relationship with food. Read on for how!

What should I be eating?

"What's the best diet to follow?" Ask this question on Dr Google, and you'll no doubt come up with millions of opinions. Eat Keto, some health gurus tout. No, Paleo is the best diet on earth! Others will say: Vegan all the way. Or the Mediterranean diet. Or the GAPs Diet. Or the Low FODMAP Diet. Or the Intermittent Fasting Diet. It's no wonder so many people are confused about what to eat.

What should you be eating? My answer: it depends.

I know, it might sound like a cop-out. But honestly, every person is different. Every person has their own bio-individuality. Some people feel better eating low-carb, while others do well with plant-based. What you need to eat to restore your body and maintain health will change overtime, depending on what body system imbalances you have, how much stress you're under, your genes, and even what season you're in.

That said, if we have a new client starting with us, I will always advise starting broad and general first. It's pretty simple: ditch the man-made processed crap, and eat more whole foods. I believe a healthy body should be able to eat all healthy, whole foods. Don't get caught up on if you should or shouldn't be eating grains because you heard they are "bad" for you, or if you should be avoiding nightshades, or legumes, or eggs. Start broad, eating high-quality whole foods first, and see how you feel. Most of the time people feel pretty darn good! And if you don't, stay tuned for the next section on healing diets.

Here's a breakdown of what whole foods actually look like. Where possible, it's best to purchase non-GMO, organic, spray-free and free-range produce. And if you're not feeling so good eating grains, legumes or nuts, try soaking and sprouting them first. If you ethically choose not to eat animal products, eat liberally from the other whole foods.

WHOLE FOODS TO EAT:

- All fruits, vegetables, herbs and spices
- All legumes
- All grains, except processed wheat
- All nuts and seeds
- All non-pasteurised dairy products
- Eggs, meat and offal
- Butter, ghee, duck fat, lard
- Cold-pressed olive oil, nut oils, coconut oil, flaxseed oil, hempseed oil, fish oil
- Water, herbal teas, kombucha, water kefir

Do I have to eat like this all the time?
This is the number one question I get asked by clients. The answer: it depends (gah, that annoying answer again!). Some people will need to eat 100% whole foods, 100% of the time while healing the body. If you consume a processed, junky meal or snack and your symptoms flare up (i.e. you get diarrhoea after eating fish and chips, or you feel depressed after eating sugar), it's best not to deviate. At least while your body is healing. Most people find they can tolerate the occasional processed meal or snack when their body systems are healed. But until that time, stay clear of reactive foods.

On the other hand, if you're someone who is *not* overly reactive to foods, you are more likely to to get away with eating off-plan occasionally (1-3 meals/snacks a week), even during your healing phase. If you feel like you can "eat anything" because processed foods don't effect how you feel, I would still encourage you to follow the whole food guidelines 100% of the time, for at least 2-4-weeks. You might be surprised by subtle (or even dramatic) changes to things like energy levels, mental clarity, mood and skin. And if no changes, then you could live by the 100% perfect, 80-90% of the time rule, where you're eating clean, whole foods most of the time to support general healing of the body, but with room to have that occasional processed meal/snack.

Do I have to make everything from scratch?
This is another common question, especially from working mums who are short on time. I mentioned earlier when I first started my healing journey that I started making everything from scratch. The thing is, I had a lot more time and less money back then. Now I run a thriving health practice, and I would rather spend my spare time with my family - rather than in the kitchen. I still make the bulk of our meals from scratch, but all the other bits and pieces - bread, granola, lunchbox snacks, sauerkraut, kombucha, healthy treats, coconut yogurt - I mostly buy packaged from reputable whole food brands.

The misconception with eating whole foods is that anything in a packet is "evil." This is not always the case. There are so many healthy whole food options now that come in a packet or jar (like my all-time grain-free Primal Alternative bakery goods - check out p.217 for more info about Primal Alternative). You just need to learn to read the ingredients. If you see ingredients that align with the whole food list above, you know you're onto a winner. Be wary of ingredients that have numbers or complicated names you can't pronounce. I've created a list of Filly-approved packaged products, which you can download from my book's website - www.chrisandfilly.fm/book

What if I react to foods on the "whole foods to eat" list?

You may have looked at the "whole foods to eat" list and saw a bunch of foods you struggle to eat. Maybe they were legumes or grains, or specific vegetables or fruits like onion or watermelon. Any negative food reaction you experience is causing inflammation – yes, even "healthy" foods can cause inflammation in susceptible people. The food itself is not the issue per se – the real issue lies within body system imbalances, especially in the gut, like pathogen overgrowth, leaky gut, SIBO or digestive organ issues, and also nervous system dysregulation. And while healing the body systems is imperative to improving tolerance to all whole foods, I do advise avoiding any reactive foods in the initial healing phase, as you want to control all possible sources of inflammation, to allow your body to heal. This is where advancing to a more restrictive short-term healing diet may be necessary.

When to use a healing diet – Hazel's story

Hazel, as you know, was struggling big time with gut issues. And when it came to eating…well, let's just say her eating patterns were all over the place. Before her gut issues flared up, she lived off convenience foods. Whatever she could grab on her lunch break (a toastie, a kebab), or on her way home from work for dinner (pizza, Mr Spud, KFC). It was no wonder her gut felt miserable, what with all the processed junk she had been consuming, as well as constantly eating on the run.

"Hazel," I said when we first met. "Let's start basic with dietary changes. Let's just cut out the processed junk, first, and see if your bloating and loose stools improve?"

I was pretty confident Hazel would come back a couple of weeks later and shower me with kisses for "fixing" her gut.

"How you feeling, Hazel?" I asked at our next treatment review.

"Terrible!" she cried. "I've pretty much been 100% - it's killing me by the way, I'm dying for some Cadbury's chocolate! - and I feel *worse*."

I sat back. I wasn't expecting this. "Oh, really? How do you feel worse?"

"My gut feels angrier - it's not just bloated, it's burning as well. And I'm sooooo itchy! My skin, my face, my eyes. I feel like clawing myself!"

I quizzed Hazel on what she had been eating, especially foods that hadn't been a big part of her previous diet. Eggs had become her go-to breakfast, and she'd been snacking on heaps on nuts and raspberries, and had even replaced her daily soft drink with kombucha.

"I think you have a histamine intolerance," I said to Hazel.

She looked at me as if I speaking latin. "Say what?"

In addition to having adrenal fatigue, SIBO and high levels of inflammation, Hazel had also developed histamine intolerance. The itchiness and burning gut with the increase of histamine foods, were a clear giveaway. Histamine is a natural chemical that is produced in your body. It also occurs in many foods like eggs, fermented foods, nuts and berries. Histamine isn't bad, but if certain body systems become imbalanced - like the adrenals, gut or detox pathways - your body starts producing too much histamine, and/or you struggle to clear histamine. Add in foods high in histamine, and you can become very symptomatic - like itchy, inflamed Hazel.

For patients like Hazel, who feel worse on a general whole food diet, or reactive to specific "healthy" foods, I will usually transition them to an elimination healing diet. Elimination diets take out further reactive foods that are high in naturally-occurring chemicals like histamine, salicylates, sulfur and oxalates. They are used short-term only, while we heal body systems and address root-causes. The goal is to always get you back to eating a wide and varied whole food diet.

Now Hazel also had SIBO, which requires a special way of eating to help reduce bacterial overgrowth. When it comes to therapeutically healing body systems, using a short-term healing diet may also be necessary. If a client has SIBO, I will prescribe them a SIBO diet which takes out high fermentable carbohydrates, like onion, potato and apples, for a short time. Healing the adrenals involves taking out major inflammatory foods like gluten, soy, processed foods, alcohol and caffeine, while also focusing on stabilising blood sugar levels with meal timing and balancing macronutrients in each meal. Restoring the microbiome is all about increasing the diversity of plant-foods. While supporting the rhythm of your sex hormones can be magnified by using different types of seeds in the luteal and follicular phases of the cycle. Doing the initial lab testing, to discover what body systems are out of balance, will help to determine and individualise the best way of eating at specific times during the healing phase.

For Hazel, we combined the SIBO diet with the low-histamine diet for a month, and she felt dramatic improvements. "I feel like a new woman!" she cried. After the initial month, and as we continued working on body systems that caused the food reactions in the first place - and the root-causes - we worked with Hazel to phase foods back in. Over the coming months she was able to transition back to a general, whole food way of eating, with very little issues.

To supplement or not to supplement

You might be wondering if doing these healing diets are enough to restore the body systems. If you've got mild, acute symptoms, a healing diet may be enough. But most women who are at a state of physiological body burnout, also need therapeutic supplement support.

I used to be in the foodie camp, the one that believed you should be able to get all your nutrients from food - food is enough to heal the body! But after my own experiences of not fully recovering from body burnout with nutrition alone, as well as doing thousands of lab tests on patients with very healthy diets, I have realised that most people need targeted supplements to physically deep heal their body systems.

The reason for this is three-fold. Firstly, sometimes your body is really failing in a specific nutrient, that you can't get in high enough doses from food alone. This might be glutathione, for example, an important antioxidant that supports detoxification. If you're glutathione levels have really flunked out, you would need to eat bucketfuls of broccoli to get the glutathione requirements needed to build your stores back up. Secondly, some people have genetic mutations, which causes their body to burn up nutrients too fast. In this case, sometimes food alone cannot support these types of defects. And thirdly (and unfortunately), our food supply isn't what it used to be, nutritionally speaking. Due to toxins in the world, our soil is not as nutrient dense as it once was, which affects the nutritional density in plant and animal foods.

I won't go into all the different supplements you need to restore body system imbalances. If you haven't done any lab testing yet, you may have the temptation to self-prescribe a bunch of supps, because you *think* you might have "adrenal fatigue" or "leaky gut." This isn't how I practice. It's always better to test, not guess. There are also so many different protocols, and to heal your body systems safely and effectively, I would always advise working with an accredited practitioner to make sure you're taking the right supplements, at the right dosages, for the right duration, and at the right time. And then of course, working on root-causes so you don't have to stay dependent on supplements to "function" and "feel good" for the rest of your life.

Finally, a note on the quality of supplements. Please - I say, please - don't go buying cheap supps from the supermarket, pharmacy or online. Quite frankly, they don't work all that well - if at all. Not only do cheap supps contain poorly absorbed nutrients (like magnesium oxide or folic acid), but they also have a lot of nasty fillers, which have no therapeutic value, and could actually be doing more harm than good. If you're using cheap supps, you'll basically be peeing your money out and doing more harm to your body, which will make the whole process far more expensive than if you invested in good-quality supplements.

Finding flow with eating - Isla's story

When it came to eating, Isla swung from eating "perfectly" to binging out on all the things. She was super self-conscious about her weight, and tried to eat a low-calorie Keto diet most of the time. But she was a sucker for cheese platters, panna cottas and bubbles and wine. And every time she indulged on these foods, the next day she'd thrash her body at the gym and eat a tight "clean" 500 calorie diet.

"I have a love-hate relationship with food," Isla said. "I'm so weak. I just can't seem to stay away from all the 'naughty' foods." She shrugged her shoulders. Hung her head. Isla was stuck in what we call the Force-Fantasy-Flounder cycle (as shown in figure 7.1):

Figure 7.1: Finding Flow

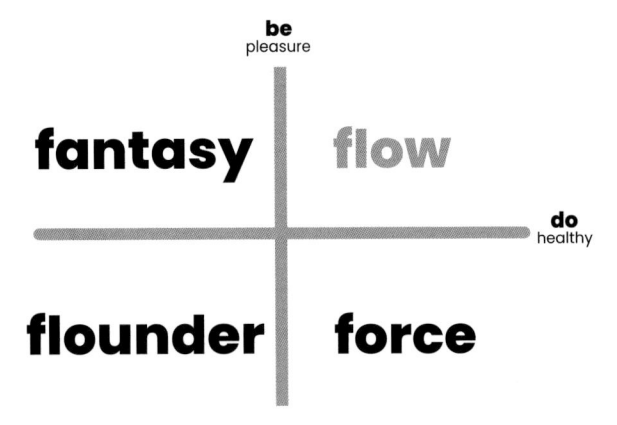

```
                    be
                  pleasure
                    |
      fantasy      |    flow
                    |
    _____|_____  do
                    |                  healthy
                    |
      flounder      |    force
                    |
```

Ultimately, you want to find flow when it comes to eating, as well as in your health and all you do in your life. Flow is the sweet spot. Flow means that you're doing the things that support health, and you're having pleasure along the way. This was definitely not Isla's experience.

Isla was forcing her clean Keto diet. While she liked eating healthy, she was constantly feeling restricted and deprived of the "naughty" foods that really gave her pleasure. Added on top of this was the need to eat healthy to lose weight. This never results in flowful eating. Forcing healthy eating purely to lose weight (or to "fix something wrong") is always driven out of fear, shame, and poor self-esteem. It shows lack of understanding of what your body and soul truly need, and also shows distrust of your body. If you force healthy eating, at some point you're going to throw it all in. This is what happened to Isla, time and time again. She reached a point of emotional pain, then swung up to fantasy-land, eating all the platters, panna cottas and bottles of wine. Fantasy is all about pleasure, fun, enjoyment - but *not* doing the things that bring you health. Shortly after Isla's fling with fun, she sunk down to floundering. Flounder is where you feel stuck, not feeling any pleasure *and* not moving towards health. For Isla, flounder was a place heavy with self-hatred, shame and guilt, and even physical pain, after giving into the damn "naughty" foods again!

Where are you when it comes to eating? Flow, force, flounder or fantasy? Understanding this cycle is incredibly important, if you're ever going to succeed in using nutrition to restore your body, regardless of if that looks like generally eating healthy, or embarking on a more restricted healing diet.

So how can you get into flow?

Eat what is right for you

Well first, you need to eat what is right for you, for where your body is at right now. There are many ways to eat healthy, and many therapeutic healing diets out there. You need to work out which one suits you based on your bio-individuality and what's going on inside your body. If you're unsure, start with ditching the processed stuff and eat more whole foods and see how you feel.

Eating rulebook

Create your own eating rulebook. Yes, there are guidelines to follow when eating healthy, and more specifically with healing diets, but you are the master of your own rulebook. If you know you'll crumble if you have to be 100% perfect, be 90% perfect (or less), and let go of any guilt or shame about not being 100% perfect.

Pleasurable eating

Next, you need to make your new way of eating pleasurable. Instead of eating foods you don't like (goodbye bland chicken breast and broccoli!), find foods within your eating plan that you not only like, but *love*! Try out new recipes or products until you find meals, snacks and healthy sweet or savoury treats that you can't wait to sink your munchers into. And find more pleasure in your every day life - beyond food. Many times women fall into emotional eating all the chocolate and icecream because they're lacking pleasure in their life.

Easy eating

Make eating easy. If it's too hard, you'll end up getting takeout. Easy for some might look like meal-prepping on a Saturday afternoon, so you have all your meals ready for your week ahead. Or following a pre-designed meal plan. Or outsourcing to a meal delivery company, or even to a local cafe to make your meals (Chris has actually done this in the past, when he was training for sports competitions and needed to eat a ton of calories!).

Cat or Salamander
Identify if you're a Cat or a Salamander. *Umm, what?* (Stay with me here!). Cats love variety and change, while Salamanders love consistency and routine. When it comes to eating, Cats love to eat different meals every day, while Salamanders are happy eating the same old foods. If you're a Cat, but you're trying to do up three bulk meals to consume for the next week, you'll lose interest pretty quick and get tempted to buy takeout! On the other hand, if you're a Salamander and you're trying to get fancy with making a new recipe every meal, you'll feel overwhelmed and stressed out, and switch back to eating convenient foods. I'm a Salamander, so I do well with making up a big dinner, which is enough for lunch and dinner the next day for the whole family, and maybe even lunch and dinner the day after that!

Eating out
Become an "eating out" health-nut. If you're a foodie like me, and love eating out at cafés, or if you travel a lot for work, eating out can be a huge sticking point. In order to find flow when eating out, do some homework on where you can eat that offers healthy *and* delicious options. I have my five or so favourite local whole food cafes that I love to eat at. When we travel for work or fun, I'll always research the best healthy places to eat, so I know I can have healthy and enjoyable food wherever I go.

Family & eating
If your kids are like mine, they can be fussy little critters. Trying to get your kids (and even partner!) on board with eating the same foods as you can be stressful. I'm a big believer that you have to fill your own cup up first, in order to give to others. Get your own eating patterns in flow first, then you'll have the tools, resources and capacity to work on the family (stay tuned for Chapter 12 - Happy Home).

Healthy relationship with food

Lastly, create a healthy relationship with your food. An unhealthy relationship often shows up as emotional eating. This could be stress eating, food addiction, anorexia, bulimia, or a dysfunctional "healthy eating" disorder. Addressing body system imbalances that can lead to emotional eating (like candida overgrowth, hormonal imbalances, depleted dopamine or vitamin B's), as well as addressing the deeper mental-emotional root-causes that we covered earlier, is where transformation happens.

Now that you're eating to support your body with the nutrients it craves, it's time to look into your sleeping patterns.

SUMMARY
RESTORATIVE NUTRITION
❼

As a summary, here's what you need to do to use nutrition to restore your body and achieve longterm healthy eating:

- Start with ditching processed foods, and eat more whole foods.
- Transition to a more structured healing diet, if you're not feeling better on a general whole food diet, or if you have specific body system imbalances that need supporting with a specific way of eating, based on lab testing.
- Incorporate high-quality, therapeutic supplements to deep heal body system imbalances, based on lab testing.
- Find flow with your eating patterns, so that you eat to support health and you're finding pleasure along the way.

CHAPTER 8

Restorative Sleep

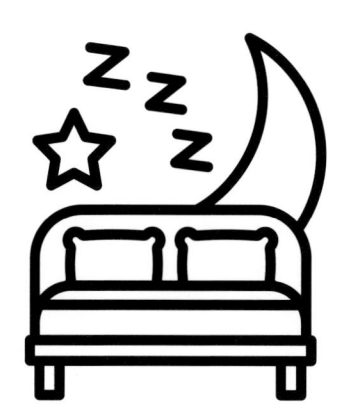

Introduction

In this chapter, you will learn all about sleep. Are your sleeping patterns healing you, or breaking you down? Is sleep contributing to your body burnout, or is body system breakdown exacerbating poor sleep? And how can you achieve a deep, restorative sleep?

    If you've ever struggled with a few nights of bad sleep (or many weeks/months/years), you'll know how crappy life can become. Poor sleep not only makes you tired and grumpy, but it's also a major cause of inflammatory conditions. This is because sleep is central to physical and mental repair. I know I suffered big time when I had babies, and I lived off broken sleep for a year straight. Then later on when COVID-19 hit, I developed periods of insomnia due to high-stress and the havoc that came from my unprocessed dysfunctional beliefs about myself. I would shake throughout the day, feel weak, achy, exhausted, on edge, and crave sugar *all the damn time* (oh the cravings!). Even my skin flared up with acne. Without a doubt, sleep was a major contributor to my own body burnout. And so, I value it highly.

After reading this chapter, you'll have a clear understanding on just how critical sleep is to healing your body (and your mind), and what you can do to bio-hack better sleep.

Sleep heals

Sleep heals. In this section, I want to show you why. Your sleep-wake cycle is governed by the sun, and your production of the hormones cortisol and melatonin (as shown in figure 8.1):

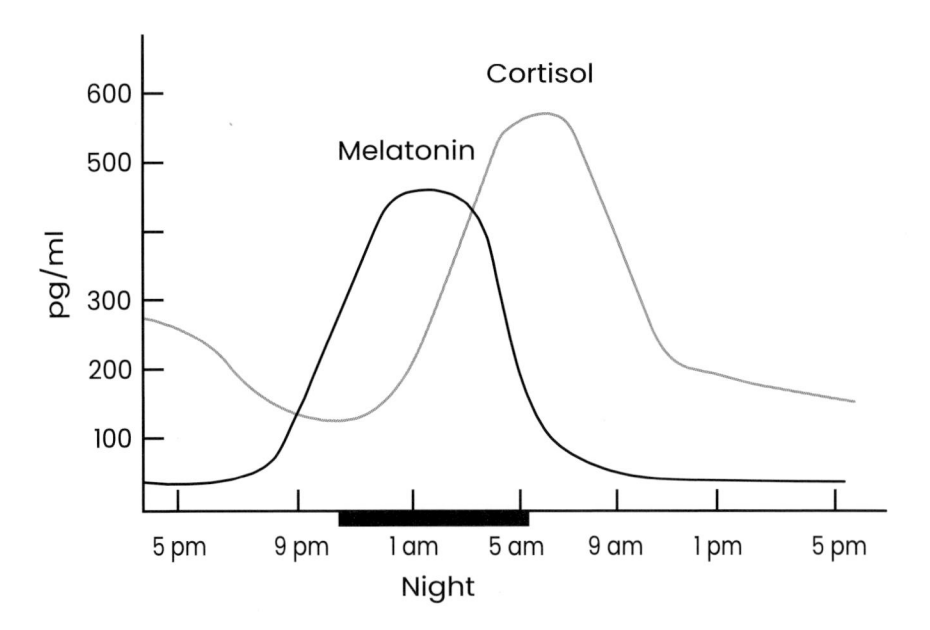

Figure 8.1: Cortisol/Melatonin Relationship

Cortisol, as you learnt in Chapter 1, is your stress hormone. It's also your rise-and-shine, get-up-and-go hormone. When the sun rises, and the light filters into your bedroom, cortisol starts to secrete, alerting you to wake up, hear the birds chirping, and excites you to start the day (if all is working functionally, that is!). Cortisol is at its highest in the morning, between 6-8am, and it slowly declines throughout the day. When the sun goes down, and cortisol is at its lowest, around 8-10pm, melatonin (your sleepy hormone) will start to secrete. Melatonin helps you to unwind, shut off, and fall to sleep. If it's being produced sufficiently, you should have a lovely, restorative, undisturbed sleep. If your mind or body is stressed-out, however, or if there are disturbances in light (not getting enough natural light in the day, or exposure to too much synthetic light at night), your melatonin production will not secrete properly, and overtime it will burnout, making it harder and harder to sleep well.

When your sleep is disrupted, major issues for your body and mind will start to arise. You see, between 10pm - 2am, your body physically repairs, and between 2am - 6am, your mind psychologically repairs from any stress or trauma it experienced that day, as documented in Paul Chek's book *How To Eat, Move & Be Healthy*. If you're going to bed too late or if you struggle to fall asleep, your body systems struggle to repair sufficiently. Likewise, if you're waking up in the early morning and struggling to fall back to sleep, or if you're getting up super early to work or exercise, psychological repair can falter.

Moral of the story is that sleep matters. Going to bed on time, being able to fall asleep, and staying asleep for the right amount of time, is absolutely essential when it comes to ending your body burnout and having optimal energy and a happier mood.

The "Light Age" - Rose's story

"How's your sleep?" I asked Rose, in our first session together.

"Not great. But I know it's my own fault. I just get so sucked into watching Netflix!"

Ah, the good old Netflix-vs-Sleep dilemma!

Rose was so exhausted by the end of the day, that she could've nodded off to sleep quite easily. But the thing was, she was sucked emotionally dry, doing everything for everyone else, that by the time the kids got to bed and the house cleaned, she desperately craved "me-time." Her "me-time" of choice: Netflix. Finally she could escape from her motherhood martyrdom (which, remember, stemmed from her deepest self-belief that she was unlovable). But by watching Netflix late at night, and dishonouring her body, she was yet again projecting her belief that she was not worthy of loving.

"I tell myself every night I'm going to watch only one episode. But they keep sucking me in. Sometimes I don't go to sleep until midnight."

Late nights. Bright screens. All of these were contributing to Rose's ongoing fatigue, brain fog and mental lethargy. How were her body systems going to ever heal without adequate sleep?

Rose is not alone. You might be cringing a little, thinking of your own nighttime bright-screen habits. You know how there was the "Ice Age" and the "Dark Ages"? Well I call our modern world the "Light Age." We literally live in a world that is full of artificial light, 24/7. Take Las Vegas, for example. That city doesn't sleep! It's full of so many lights, that even migratory birds lose their bearings. While being exposed to lots of light during the day is beneficial for our sleep-wake cycle, blue light creeping into our homes and workplaces at night, are really stuffing up our body clocks.

"Rose," I said. "Did you know that every time you switch your iPad on to watch Netflix at night, your brain thinks it is the sun rising? Same as if you're working late on the computer, flicking through Instagram on your phone, or watching TV, or if you have lots of bright lights inside your home or street lamps shining into your bedroom."

Rose nodded slowly, the penny dropping. "Right...So every time my brain sees light at night, it gets confused about what time of day it is?"

"Correct," I said. "And when the brain sees blue-light, cortisol will peak, which suppresses melatonin. Even if you fall asleep ok after you switch Netflix off, you're never going to get restorative sleep because your hormones get all mixed up. In actual fact, cortisol can take *hours* to clear from your blood stream."

There's a crazy study, in Linda Geddes book, *Chasing the Sun*, that even showed that a tiny torch, shone under the blanket onto participants' legs, was enough light to increase cortisol and disrupt melatonin production.

But it's not just electronic lights that we're more exposed to. Many high-achieving, busy women are also far less exposed to the sunlight, with many work and domestic hours occurring in doors. Our bodies were designed to live in natural light during the day. By design, this supports melatonin production later at night. Some experts, like T.S. Wiley in *Lights Out*, argue that this combination of more electronic light at night, with less natural sunlight is the root-cause for many health conditions, such as cardiovascular disease, cancer, diabetes, depression.

Bio-hack your sleep-wake cycle by harnessing the power of light

So does this mean you need to live like a caveman? Bunker down in darkness, as soon as the sun goes down? Fortunately, you can still be an adult and stay up after sunset, *and* improve your sleep-wake cycle, by following these bio-hacking light tips. These are especially important to trial, if you struggle with sleep, or if you're sleeping, but not sure if it's restorative sleep.

- Turn off bright-lights and screens at least 1hr before bed.
- If you choose to use screens at night, reduce the damaging effects by using blue-light blocking devices (i.e. glasses, screen blockers). Also reduce the brightness of your phone, tablet and computer.
- Replace all CFLs (compact fluorescent light bulbs) with incandescent light bulbs, or minimally LEDs.
- After sunset, try to use dimmer lights, lamps, or even go "antique" with candles.
- Harness the power of the sun. Sleep expert, Michael Breus, says that getting outside in the morning for at least 15 minutes (even on cloudy days), and again for an hour or two in the afternoon before sunset, is the best medicine for resetting your sleep-wake cycle.

- If doing the above points don't help you to fall asleep and stay asleep, we've created a more advanced 3-Day Sleep Detox protocol which can help even stubborn insomnia. Basically all lights and electronics are turned off after the sun goes down, and you live in candlelight only. Our family have done this a few times, and the results are mind-blowing! Our oldest daughter has always been a night owl, and struggles to fall asleep early (some nights it's 10pm!). When we do the 3-Day Sleep Detox, she's sound asleep by 7:30pm. I also have the deepest sleeps when doing the 3-Day Sleep Detox and wake up buzzing with energy. Go to my book's website to download the protocol - www.chrisandfilly.fm/book
- Your bedroom environment matters too. Stay tuned for Chapter 10 - Home Set Up.

Finding your ideal sleep pattern

So how long should you be sleeping? This is a super common question I get asked. The National Sleep Foundation will give you a standard answer of 7 - 9 hours.

But I want to help you discover your own ideal sleep pattern.

While there's a general time-frame for optimal sleep (i.e. 10pm - 6am), this can vary for people due to their individual genetic variances and biological clocks. For example, one person will feel better going to bed earlier and waking up earlier (i.e. 9pm - 5am), while another person will feel their best going to bed later and waking up later (i.e. 11pm - 7am). The ideal duration for sleep also differs for each individual. One person may need 9 hours of sleep every night to feel restored (this is me!), while another person will feel good on 7 or 8 hours of sleep (my husband Chris feels best with 7 hours of sleep - 8 or 9 hours of sleep makes him feel sluggish and tired).

Dr Michael Breus in his book *The Power of When*, goes even further in showing that there are four distinct chronotypes:

Lion - ideal wake time is 6am, ideal sleep time is 10pm.
Bear - ideal wake time is 7am, ideal sleep time is 11pm.

Wolf - ideal wake time is 9am, ideal sleep time is 1am.
Dolphin - ideal wake time is 6:30am, ideal sleep time is 11:30pm.

What's most important is that you go to sleep and wake up at the *same time*. Having a regular sleep/wake time will help restore your circadian rhythm and promote a restorative sleep.

Here's how to identify your own ideal sleep pattern:

Track using an app
There are sleeping apps (i.e. Pillow app) which can track your sleep with fairly good accuracy. It monitors your movement, noise and breathing patterns while you sleep, and can identify if you are getting good quality sleep by measuring your 4 Stages of Sleep (i.e. transitional/light sleep, rapid-eye-movement sleep, and deep sleep). After taking measurements over multiple nights, it can then predict your best bed time for optimal sleep, and also how long you need to sleep.

Alarm clock method
If you're not an "app" person, this is also an effective (and easy) method to identify your ideal sleep pattern. Start by choosing a time to go to bed (i.e. 10pm, or based on what you think your chronotype is) and go to bed at the same time every night. If you wake up a few minutes before your alarm, you have found your ideal sleep time. If you're waking up to your alarm, try going to bed 20min earlier each night until you find your ideal bedtime.

Note: this method will only work if you are going to sleep and staying asleep relatively well (and if your kids are no longer waking!).

Hazel's sleep success
Hazel, as you most likely remember, was addicted to work. Her big issue when it came to sleep was being able to switch off her computer at a decent hour. She got lost in her to-do list after the boys went to bed, and sometimes it was 2am when she realised the time. Her body was flooding with cortisol, what with the late night exposure to blue-light and her mind in an alerted work-

mode. By the time she stumbled to bed, her brain was in overdrive, racing, anxious thoughts trying to problem-solve, and she struggled to fall asleep.

During a group coaching session, we worked with Hazel to create an evening routine. Hazel discovered her ideal sleep time was 11pm, and so we worked backwards to create an evening schedule that would lead to better sleep patterns. She would come home from work at 6pm to a dinner made by her Nanny, which she would eat with her boys. Her boys would have a shower, PJ's, and then they would play a game or read some books together as a family. The boys would go to bed by 8pm, and this would give Hazel an hour to finish up any work. She would wear blue-light blocking glasses as she worked, and would turn off the computer when the alarm went off at 9pm. The alarm was important, otherwise Hazel would get lost in her work. At 9pm, she would potter around, doing house chores that needed to be done. And then by 10pm she was in bed with a novel, giving herself space to wind down before sleep.

Hazel struggled with implementing this evening routine initially. She felt antsy, even anxious, doing "less" in the evening. This wasn't a surprise, considering her over-working patterns came from a deep, unconscious fear of being inadequate. If this belief was never uncovered or reframed, doing "less" and living "slower" would feel unsafe. As Hazel worked on her self-limiting beliefs (a great reframe for Hazel was "it's safe to be slow" and "I am more than adequate exactly as I am"), she was able to let go of her workaholic patterns, and start behaving in a self-loving and self-healing way. She started to consistently go to bed on time, and with the help of her inner healing work, and her adrenal supplement protocol, her mind began to feel calmer, and she was able to fall asleep without the to-do list racing in her mind.

Now just a final note before we put this sleep chapter to bed (pun intended!). If you have read this chapter and you feel like you've done all the sleep hygiene bio-hacking out there, and you can honestly say you are giving yourself permission to be healthy, and not forcing it, yet you still struggle to get your forty winks, there may be some body system imbalances directly affecting your sleep patterns. Just like Hazel, you may need some lab-based therapeutic supplemental support, to reset body systems - like your adrenals, brain chemicals, sex hormones or detox pathways - that can impair a good night's sleep. I have seen dramatic changes in insomniac clients even after a few weeks of starting on protocols. In fact, the number one improvement when a patient first starts working with us is, hands-down, better sleep!

Now that you're sleeping to support your body and your health, it's time to look into restorative movement.

SUMMARY
RESTORATIVE SLEEP

As a summary, here's what you need to do to achieve deep sleep to restore your body:

- Utilise the power of light to bio-hack your sleep-wake cycle. More natural light during the day, less artificial light at night.
- Discover your own ideal sleep pattern, and aim to go to sleep and wake up the same time every day.
- Create your own evening routine that leads to optimal sleep and health.
- Get to the root of your dysfunctional beliefs to support a calm mind, so you can feel safe to sleep.
- If you're doing all of the above, and you're still struggling to sleep. Test and therapeutically recorrect any body systems that can affect sleep.

CHAPTER 9
Restorative Movement

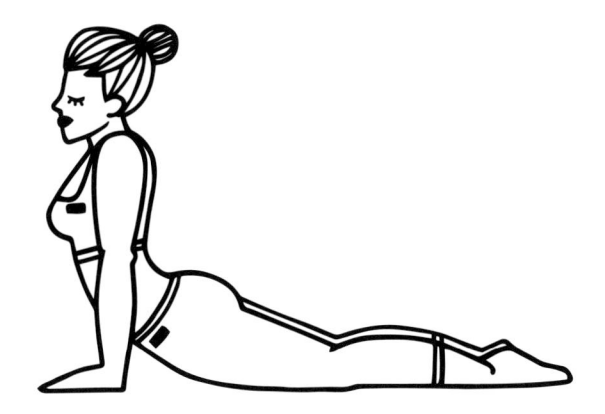

Introduction
In this chapter, you will learn all about movement. But don't expect this chapter to be only about "exercise." Movement is far more than just hitting the gym for a workout. In this chapter, I look into whether your movement patterns are supporting your body, or in actual fact, breaking it down.

The thing is, movement - or lack there of - can contribute to body burnout. On one hand, there are plenty of studies that show full well that sedentary living leads to disease, including mental ill health. And this is very prevalent - one third of the global population engages in insufficient physical activities. As a busy, high-achieving woman, I know it can be tricky to "fit" exercise in amongst all of the other responsibilities. On the opposite end of the spectrum, however, there are also plenty of women over-exercising, which is also negatively impacting body systems. This might not necessarily look like training at the gym two times a day or running ultramarathons. An average woman could be doing a HIIT workout three times a week, or even a daily 1 hour walk, and still be "over-exercising" if the movement is too intense for the current state of her body, or if her body is not recovering properly. Restorative movement also relates to the movement and flow within your body. Are your bowels moving properly, are your detox pathways flowing? Or is there stagnation and blockages affecting your health?

After reading this chapter, you'll have a clear understanding of how movement can either heal or damage the body systems, as well as how to use movement to restore (rather than cause more damage to) your body, specifically for where you're at right now.

Movement and body systems

Just like nutrition, many mums are confused about what type of exercise they should be doing, especially when they're feeling tired, inflamed and burned-out. Are HIIT classes ok? Should I still be training for that half-marathon? Is yoga enough to keep me fit and healthy? How many steps should I be doing? Am I going to put on weight if I reduce the intensity of exercise to heal? Exercise is a stressor. It's a good stressor in that it can help you to get stronger, fitter and leaner. But you can only handle so much if you're in a burned-out state. Too much, and it can burn you out further. In this chapter, I want to help you identify what type of movement is right for you. Understanding exactly where your body systems are at can determine what type of movement you need to heal, the intensity you can handle in your present state, and what nutrients you need to support recovery from exercise, so that movement is healing, rather than damaging.

Adrenals - Hazel

Hazel was in early stages of adrenal fatigue. For Hazel, adding in exercise was beneficial, as she needed to "burn-off" excess cortisol that was being pumped through her bloodstream. Hazel's movement prescription: get off your butt Hazel and exercise daily, especially the aerobic type like a brisk walk, jog, swim, bike ride or gym class.

If Hazel's adrenal results, however, had showed later stages of adrenal fatigue and depletion, adding in huffy-puffy exercise would have been an extra stressor that her adrenals just couldn't handle. In this case, I would've still encouraged daily exercise, but low-intensity movement like walking, swimming, yoga and stretching. And as energy levels and resilience increase, so too would the intensity of exercise increase.

Brain - Rose

It's common knowledge that physical movement can lift mood. You've no doubt experienced this after going for a brisk walk along the beach. We've even had patients claim that exercise worked better than anti-depressant medication. And while I'd always encourage incorporating movement into your lifestyle for mental health, over-exercising can lead to neurotransmitter depletion.

Rose's dopamine levels had depleted. And while there were many root-causes that lead to this, over-exercising was likely a contributor. Rose had been an avid exerciser prior to having kids. She loved getting the feel-good dopamine hit that exercise brings! But, overtime, this dopamine hit became an addiction, and she exercised far more than what is balanced and healthy. The more you indulge in addictive habits, the more your dopamine depletes.

If your labs are showing up with low brain chemicals, especially dopamine and adrenaline/noradrenaline, be wise with how you're using exercise, and get clear on *why* you're using it.

Mitochondria - Rose

Rose also had mitochondrial issues, which also compounded her ability to exercise. The mitochondria are stimulated when you move and oxygenate your body and muscle tissue through exercise. In this regard, movement is critical for the health of your mitochondria and production of ATP energy. However, if the mitochondria have become damaged - like in Rose's case - exercise can cause further damage. You see, when you exercise, your mitochondria produces ATP energy, which also spits off free-radicals. This is a normal physiological response, and your antioxidant nutrients should come along and mop up free-radicals. However, if your body is in a state of inflammation, which is often the case when the mitochondria are damaged, those free-radicals can turn back onto the mitochondria, and cause *further* damage. This is the number one reason why Rose felt even *more* fatigued after exercise, even after a short walk around her farm, rather than energised.

Rose still needed to move. Not moving would also cause damage to the mitochondria. The challenge for Rose was to gradually increase her exercise intensity, so that she never felt "wasted" after a movement session. Using breath-work to oxygenate her mitochondria was also critical in rebuilding her mitochondria, especially in the earlier stages when she wasn't yet ready for more huffy-puffy aerobic exercise. Every month Rose felt a 10% improvement in her energy levels and stamina, and by 9-months she was easily (and mindfully!) doing 5-10km jogs and pilates workouts at home.

GI System - Hazel
Restorative movement isn't just about exercise and moving your limbs. It's also about how well your organs are flowing. Hazel's gut was not moving optimally. The fact that she alternated between constipation and diarrhoea, and constantly felt bloated, was a clear sign. Your GI system needs to flow in two major ways. First, it needs to produce and secrete digestive juices, to help breakdown foods and keep them moving through your GI tract. And secondly, your gut motility needs to be in tip-top shape, to contract and move food (and microbes) from one end to the other.

Alongside therapeutic support for SIBO, we also prescribed Hazel some specific gut movement exercises to retrain her GI tract to proper functioning. Hazel started performing a special diaphragmatic breathing technique which massages the colon, to stimulate motility. You can see a video on my book's website

- [www.chrisandfilly.fm/book.](www.chrisandfilly.fm/book) She also included rebounding (jumping on an exercise trampoline) into her daily exercise regime, and used a stool to elevate her knees when she went to the toilet, to support healthy bowel movements. I also encouraged Hazel to take five deep belly breaths before eating each meal, to switch her body into a relaxed state, so that her digestive organs could start secreting digestive juices again. And chew, Hazel, chew! Hazel slowed down her eating habits, and chewed her food 10-20 times before swallowing, to support better GI functioning.

Detox System - Isla
Just like the gut, your detox system needs to "move" to clear nasty toxins and excess hormones from the body. Your liver first needs to break down toxins ready for excretion, then you need to move those toxins out of your body through the bowels, kidneys and skin pores. Issues can arise if either the liver is sluggish, or if there are blockages in the eliminatory pathways.

    Isla's detox pathways weren't flowing sufficiently. Her liver had burned-out, and she wasn't producing enough bile to properly send toxins and excess oestrogen into the gut, ready to poo out. Part of Isla's movement prescription was to back off on her intense gym workouts, to allow her nutrients that support detoxification to replenish. She also added in detox-supporting techniques, especially when we started working on her bile production and detox pathways. Increasing water intake was number one, to help flush out toxins and excess hormones. She also got her sweat on with regular saunas and hot epsom salt baths, to really open up her eliminatory pathways and support lymphatic drainage. And she worked her way up to hot-cold shower therapy, to help stimulate her detox pathways and nervous system.

Start with steps

After reading all of that, you might be wondering where you should start with your own movement program, especially if you haven't done functional lab tests to pin-point where your body systems are at. Lady, if you're reading this, I'm assuming you're feeling pretty burned-out. If this is you and you're currently sedentary, I would say start with steps. Or, if you're on the opposite side of the spectrum, and you're still pushing it with intense exercise, I would also say, back off, slow down, and start with steps.

Walking is the backbone of health. It's what our bodies were designed to do. Our ancient ancestors weren't sitting around on stones all day. They walked as they hunted, gathered, and moved from one landmark to the next. Primal enthusiast, Mark Sisson, says hardly anybody walks as much as what they should. Walking is a low-intensity, safe place to start (or to drop back down to) if you're in a state of body-burnout.

So how much walking should you be doing a day? Data suggests that 10,000 steps a day is a good goal for optimal health. It's estimated that the average adult takes around 3,000 - 4,000 steps per 30 minute walk. And that a sedentary adult usually takes about 3,000 - 4,000 steps per day. If you're currently sedentary, sitting at the desk all day working, with minimal movement around your office and at home, you'll need to start adding in a daily walk of 30-60 minutes. If you feel "time-poor" you can do these walks in 10 minute chunks, or walk while you're doing another task. Can you do some phone calls while you walk around the block for 10 minutes? Or can you wander for 30 minutes while you're eating your lunch? Can you get more active with the kids, when you take them to activities?

You might be thinking: *But what if I'm so exhausted, that even a 20minute walk wastes me?* If this is you, baby steps. Do only what you can - it might only be 2,000 steps a day - and slowly build up to 10,000 steps.

When to increase exercise intensity

If you're struggling to exercise because what you're doing is exhausting you (even if it is just walking), or if you feel like you're ready to increase the intensity of exercise, but not sure how to do it safely, this section will help you out. Let me introduce you to the concept of Graded Exercise Therapy (GET).

GET's original usage is for treatment of chronic fatigue, as documented in Toby Morrison's book *Chronic Fatigue Syndrome*. It involves gentle physical activity which is introduced gradually. As you gain strength and energy, the intensity of physical exertion is slowly increased over time, to produce an adaptation in your body, so that you can grow fitter and stronger - and start thriving. This form of therapy is highly controlled, and to be done correctly, it has to be followed according to a strict, balanced exercise plan, which includes mandatory periods of rest. The main aim is not to overexercise and not to push the body to its limits, which would be detrimental to your health. This type of therapy can be efficient in alleviating fatigue, disturbed sleep, low mood, anxiety, pain, and other symptoms related to body burnout. It's a great tool to use if lab results are showing later stages of adrenal fatigue, mitochondrial dysfunction, and liver detoxification issues.

GET involves doing a pushing exercise (like wall, knee or floor pushups), a squatting exercise (like a hand assisted squat, air squat or weighted squats), a core exercise (like dead bugs, sit-ups or V-ups) and an aerobic exercise (like walking, jogging, cycling or swimming). Depending on where you're at vitality and active-wise, will depend on what level of exercise you do, and the duration of repetitions. You start with a baseline of exercises that feel "easy" and repeat those exercises for 2-weeks. You will know if you can increase the intensity of the exercise if:

- You feel like your exercise is doing nothing for you and it's far too easy.
- You have maintained your health (haven't gotten worse) after exercising consistently for 2-weeks.
- You have increased in energy consistently for 2-weeks (not in ebbs or flows).

- Your muscles don't get tired or sore after or during exercise (you want to feel it a little bit).

If you have your own exercise regime - whether that be with a personal trainer, gym class, pilates sessions, or even just your daily walks - you can use the same points above to assess if you are doing too much, too soon.

Movement and the mindset shift

If you're an avid exerciser and you've been feeling a bit anxious reading this chapter, thinking: *how can I give up my CrossFit classes or Bootcamps?!* (even though you secretly know it's burning you out), I see you. This mindset shift around exercise was something I struggled with, big time. In fact, I struggled with it so much that it took me *years* to finally honour my body, stop, slow down, and pivot to movement that was restorative, rather than damaging.

Prior to setting up our functional medicine practice, Chris was a personal trainer and strength and conditioning coach. He owned a gym, and I was his most diligent student. Always showing up to his Bootcamp and CrossFit classes. Before kids, I trained everyday - sometimes twice a day. I was fast and strong and fit. I could do 100+ pushups without stopping. 20+ pull-ups without a break. But when I started having babies, and my health fell apart, so did my physical prowess. I struggled to run. I trembled as I tried to do one pushup. I kept getting sick after intense workouts. Yet still I kept on pushing my body, trying to "do" what I used to be able to do. Until one day, when I attempted a kettlebell deadlift, I heard my lower back crack. For 18-months I lived with chronic sciatica pain, sometimes so bad I couldn't get out of bed. And even then, I kept pushing my body in the gym on the days I felt "ok." It always ended badly. I knew deep in my heart that I was hurting my body with exercise, that I was preventing it from healing. Yet my mind kept saying: *No! You used to be able to do this. You should be able to do it now!* I was trying to chase that "fit girl" back in the past. And I was also secretly scared that if I stopped exercising intensely, I would stack on weight.

The pain eventually stacked up enough that I knew I had to change. I finally acknowledged that all the supps in the world, and all the healthy foods, were not going to deep heal my body systems, if I constantly stressed out my body with the wrong type of exercise. It required a huge mindset shift to let go of that "fit girl" from the past. But it was made possible because I created such a compelling vision of who I wanted to become - a loving mother and wife, a practitioner that walks the talk, a woman that is deeply connected to herself - and worked through self-limiting beliefs that caused me to cling onto the "fit girl" in the first place. And guess what? Not only did my body heal, but I didn't put on any weight. In fact, I looked more toned because there was far less inflammation in my body. At the time of writing this, I continue to exercise slower - walking, swimming, yoga, playing with the kids and puppy, occasional long hikes - and my body feels the best it has ever felt, and still no extra weight.

If you're in a state of body burnout, and you need to change up your exercise regime to heal (whether that be dropping the intensity, or moving more) but you're feeling yourself resisting, here are some questions to ponder:

- What are your thoughts when it comes to exercise?
- What are the stories that you tell yourself about exercise? Are they things like:
  - No pain, no gain.
  - Quitters are losers.
  - I have to feel dead to know I had a good workout.
  - I need to sweat to lose weight.
  - I'm too fat to exercise.
  - I don't have time to exercise.
  - I don't like the way exercise makes me feel.
- What mantras do you say to yourself over and over again, that may not be serving you?
- What are you trying to prove with exercise?
- Are you honouring your body with movement? If not, why not?

Whatever your non-serving story is, there's going to be internal friction if you need to change what you're currently doing. Get clear on your vision again, reprogram self-limiting beliefs, adult up and give yourself permission and safety to experience something different.

Now that you've nailed restorative movement for where you're currently at, it's time to move to the final part of this book - Step Four: Heal Thy Environment.

SUMMARY
RESTORATIVE MOVEMENT

As a summary, here's what you need to do to create your own movement regime that will restore your body, not break it down:

- Get clear on where your body systems are at with lab testing, and tailor movement of the limbs and organs for where you're at right now.
- Keep it simple, and start with steps. Either increase your daily steps if you are currently sedentary, or drop back high intensity exercise to daily steps as a baseline.
- Use GET techniques to know when you are exercising safely, and when you can increase intensity.
- Continue with your inner mind work, if you're resisting implementing a new movement regime.

STEP FOUR
Heal Thy Environment

STEP FOUR
HEAL THY ENVIRONMENT

In Step Four: Heal Thy Environment, I go over the final step of ending your body burnout, and that is healing your environment. You are, after all, a product of your environment. You do not live in isolation. Your mind and your body are constantly interacting with things in your environment (for better or for worse). To fully unravel yourself from all the sticky root-causes that are holding you back from truly shining, you must now look outwards, and into your environment.

In Step Four, I go over three important aspects of your environment that could be leading to body burnout, or preventing you from healing, and they are: home setup, toxin-free home and happy home. Is your home setup sabotaging your good intentions, or is it supporting your self-honouring mindset and new behaviours? Are there hidden toxins stressing out your system, or do you live in a clean, healthy space conducive for healing? Are your relationships at home triggering negative emotions or behaviour, or is your new-found love and respect for yourself naturally flowing into your family?

CHAPTER 10

Home Setup

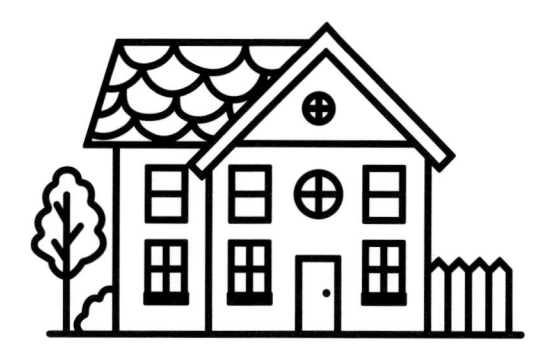

Introduction
In this chapter, we're going to pull everything that you have learned so far about healing your mind and body, and make sure your environment is setup for successful implementation.

    The way your home is set up, is going to make or break your healing outcomes. Chris and I were talking about ideas for this chapter at the time of writing this book, and overhearing us my nine year old daughter chimed in, very profoundly: "Mum, Dad. Your home is a reflection of your mind, and how you think and feel." Yes Poppy, it sure is! Your environment is an outward reflection of your internal commitment to your health and ending your body burnout.

What you value will always show up in your environment. If you're one foot in, one foot out, it will be evident in your kitchen cupboards, your bedroom, your workspace. When you embark on a life changing experience, there will always be teething issues initially, as you try to shift your inner landscape, learn new ways of eating, respond to stressors, engage in healing movement. But if your environment continues to stay disorganised, chaotic, painful or down-right sabotaging, it's going to make implementing the healthy things super difficult. And to be frank, your new habits and lifestyle just won't stick. Which will only ever lead to short-term improvements (if any) of your symptoms, leaving you frustrated, in pain and back at square one. Mark Caine says: "the first secret to success is when you refuse to be a captive of the environment in which you find yourself. James Clear in *Atomic Habits* also emphasises that setting up your environment is a key factor in creating new habits. Lovely, it's time to take back your power, get clear on your values and recommit to your vision, and create an environment that is healing, not destructing.

After reading this chapter, you'll have some really practical steps to make sure key areas of your home and workplace are set up for success and sustainable health and wellbeing. These areas are your kitchen, bedroom and office setup.

Kitchen setup - Isla's story

Ok, let's get practical. Let's transform your kitchen! In Chapter 7, we looked into Restorative Nutrition. Now, you might've naturally rearranged your kitchen already, to ensure your new way of eating is a success. But if you haven't, read on.

John Berardi, PhD said: "If a food is in your possession or located in your residence, either you, someone you love, or someone you marginally tolerate will eventually eat it." How often have you started a diet and you've purchased all your healthy food, yet you were still buying processed junk food for the rest of your family? How long was it before you were tempted to the "dark side"? If you're like most people, you eventually succumbed, at some point.

Isla had tried all the diets out there. Yet as we know, she wasn't very good at sticking to a healthy and balanced way of eating, longterm. While there were deeper root-causes that she was addressing, one very simple issue was her kitchen setup. Isla continued buying chocolate and wine and cookies for her partner. She thought her "will-power" would be enough to refrain from the foods she really loved. Of course she continued yoyo-ing. As part of our holistic approach to addressing Isla's eating patterns, we got practical over a virtual coaching session, and did a kitchen makeover. We had Isla pull out all the food from her fridge and cupboards. We analysed her cooking utensils. We checked out her space to see if it was conducive for meal prepping and storing. During the session, we helped Isla ditch the bad stuff, and replace it with the good stuff. Specifically, Isla tossed out:

- Refined, packaged cookies, cakes, chips, breads, etc.
- Trans-fats - vegetable oil, canola oil, and foods containing these oils.
- Ice cream, sugar-flavoured yogurts.
- Wheat-based processed bread (i.e. white, multigrain, wholemeal, rye) and pasta.
- Sugary cereals.
- Condiments and sauces high in sugar, or that contain artificial additives (jams, savoury sauces, mayonnaise, sweet syrups).
- Alcohol, soft drink, cordial, caffeinated drinks.

And replaced these foods with the whole foods listed in Chapter 7. And after a long discussion, Isla also went on to get her partner on board with a healthier way of eating, which meant the fridge and cupboards remained stocked with healthier foods (most of the time). And as she worked on her inner healing and broke-free from self-limiting beliefs and emotional triggers around food, she found over time that she had no desire to binge out on wine and cakes and chocolate. And even when that food made its way into the house, or if she found herself at a party, she was happy with just one glass of bubbles, or a small piece of slice.

In addition to changing up the food contents in your kitchen, you'll also want to make sure your kitchen is organised, and you have all the cooking appliances to make cooking and meal prepping easy. Are you missing any appliances regularly mentioned in recipes, or that could make your cooking experience faster or easier? Would getting a fast-speed blender (like a Thermomix) to make smoothies, bliss balls or your own nut-based milk make life easier? Do you have enough saucepans or frypans, to have a few meals on the go (if you're opting for meal prepping in bulk)? Are your knives nice and sharp to make chopping effortless? Do you have food stored in an organised manner, or are food items all over the place? These might seem little, but we've had so many clients feeling blocked around cooking, and it's simply because they don't have the right equipment or their kitchen is too disorganised to work in. And in fact, research shows the messier and disorganised your kitchen, the more unhealthy the eating patterns. You also want to make sure you're using "healthy" cookware. Some cookware are coated with harmful chemicals, like teflon, that are carcinogenic. Opt for cookware that is made from cast iron, glass or stainless steel as healthier, safer options. Also avoid using aluminium foil and plastics when cooking or heating up food.

Bedroom setup

Now your kitchen is sorted, let's venture into your bedroom. In Chapter 8, I spoke all about Restorative Sleep, and ways you can enhance your sleep-wake cycle. What I didn't get into is your physical bedroom environment.

When setting up your bedroom for restorative sleep, you want to create a cave-like environment. Humans have evolved to hibernate at night, and operate best when we sleep in a cave, safe from predators, and comfortable enough to promote a restful night's sleep. Here's how to set your bedroom up like a cave:

Keep your cave DARK

As discussed in Chapter 8, artificial light at night can really screw up your sleep-wake cycle. Even when your eyes are closed, your body will respond to any light filtering onto your skin, causing a spike of cortisol, and melatonin to suppress. Make your bedroom as dark as possible, especially free of artificial light.

- Use blackout curtains if you have artificial light outside (e.g. street lights) lighting up the room.
- Disconnect digital clocks or electronic lights.
- Don't use night lamps or glowing aromatherapy diffusers.
- A sleeping mask is a simple and cost effective option, if you're travelling and sleeping in a lit-up room, or you don't want to get new curtains.

Keep your cave COOL

It's important to keep your bedroom at a comfortable temperature (15-20 degrees celsius tends to be ideal for most people). If you're too hot, melatonin production will be suppressed. If too cold, your body will be in a stressed-state.

- Seasonally switching your bedding (i.e. lighter doona cover in the summer, heavier one in the winter) will make it easier to maintain a comfortable body temperature.
- You may also need to use a fan or open up your windows if it's too hot. Natural air is better than using an artificial air conditioner every night, which can trigger allergies, respiratory issues and harbour mould.

Keep your cave CLEAN

It's important to keep the air quality clean in your bedroom, to improve oxygenation for a restful sleep. Oxygen also supports better brain health which can affect your energy and mental clarity during the day. Keeping your cave clean also means keeping it tidy.

- Air filters are the most effective option for improving air quality.
- Plants can be an inexpensive way to clean indoor air. Just make sure they are free of mould.

- Keep your bedroom tidy. A study showed that people with more mess and clutter in their bedroom, had trouble sleeping.
- Keep your bedroom sacred for sleep only (and sexy time, ha!). That means no TV-watching and no working in the bedroom. This helps condition your brain to know that when you're in your bedroom, it means sleep.

Keep your cave HEALTHY

It's important to have a sleeping surface (i.e. mattress and bedding) that is non-toxic.

- Rotate and flip your mattress every 6-months to increase the mattress life span. Regularly putting your sun out in the mattress, will also help keep it clean of nasty bugs.
- Check there is no mould at the bottom of the bed or on/in the mattress or pillows. Some people are very sensitive to mycotoxins, which can cause insomnia, and other health-related symptoms. Also check for mould on the walls, roof and windowsills.
- Change your pillow every one to two years, especially if you suffer with allergies or skin issues.

Workspace

What's your workspace looking like, these days? I lot of people post-COVID are working from home, and even if you don't, your workspace is most likely a place where you are spending a lot of your time. There are countless studies linking clutter with high levels of stress. A USA study found that levels of the stress hormone cortisol where higher in mothers whose home environment was cluttered. And likewise, stress and overwhelm follows through into a cluttered, disorganised workspace. Workspace mission number one: clean up your workspace. Creating a system where you can easily store and access resources, will take a huge stressor off your shoulders.

How you work in your environment, is also important. Let's chat ergonomics. If your workspace is set up dysfunctionally, it can lead to a world of pain. Poor ergonomics can lead to joint pain, headaches, fluid retention, irritability, anxiousness, digestive issues, and fatigue. Working long hours at a desk can take a huge toll on your body. You will want to make sure your chair is set up at the right height for your desk, and your computer is set up at the right height for your sitting position, so you don't injure your wrists, neck, hips or back. Taking regular breaks is also imperative. Dr Kristy Goodwin in her book *Dear Digital* has some fantastic micro-habits for setting up your workspace for health and productivity, and to prevent burnout.

A lot of my work is done working on the computer. Not only am I consulting a lot, and mostly virtual consults, but I'm also using the computer to create content, organise partnerships and events, and manage virtual staff. I used to sit at my desk and work, all day long, day in and day out. In the end, I ended up in a lot of pain, especially my lower back and hips, and RSI (repetitive stress injury) in my wrists. This physical pain added to my already overflowing stress bucket, which exacerbated my anxiety, energy and gut issues.

When I started my own healing journey, I knew things needed to change with how I worked. I changed my desk and chair so that it was more economically-friendly, which eased the RSI. And I made an effort to change up how I worked on the computer. On consulting days, I sat at my work desk, and on non-consulting days, I worked on my computer standing up at a high bench, or I'd take my laptop outside and work in the garden, lying down on my belly. I continue changing up my position to this day, and it works beautifully to prevent work-related pain.

Any pain is a message from your body, telling you that something is not quite right, or out of balance. It might be that your workspace ergonomics need adjusting. Or, very often, it's a sign that you're working *too* much. Listen to your pain, and figure out if it's coming from a dysfunctional set up in your environment, or a dysfunctional belief or behavioural pattern, stemming from a need to do-do-do. Your body craves health, and it will always tell you when you've broken rapport with yourself.

Now that you've got the key physical areas in your home setup, let's look at cleaning up any nasty, hidden toxins from your home.

SUMMARY
RESTORATIVE MOVEMENT
— **10** —

As a summary, here's what you need to do to set up your home for successful body system healing:

- Get your kitchen setup and organised with the right foods and cookware.
- Get your bedroom setup like a cave, to up-level your sleep.
- Get your workspace setup in an ergonomically-friendly way, and clear up clutter from your environment.

CHAPTER 11

Low Tox Home

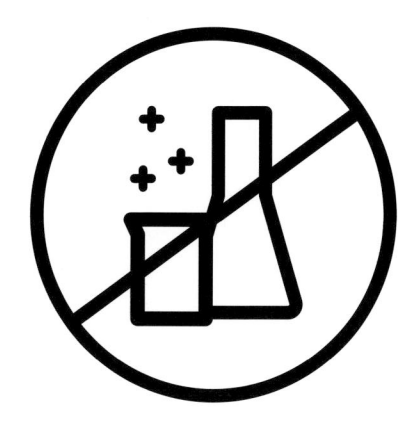

Introduction

In this chapter, you'll learn all about the different types of hidden toxins that could be lurking in your home, and causing your body systems to burnout.

Humans produce more than 250 billion tonnes of chemical substances a year. The world has never been more toxic. Dr Kalish, my first functional medicine mentor, said that in his 30 years of practice, now more than ever is he seeing clinical evidence of the damaging impact of environmental toxins on the body. I'm also seeing this in lab testing - toxins directly impacting body systems such as the adrenals, neurotransmitters, mitochondria, detox pathways, the gut and sex hormones. And research backs this up: toxins are disrupting our hormones, causing oxidative damage to our cells, and are linked to diseases like cancer, heart problems, and infertility. The prevalence of asthma and allergic diseases have also increased worldwide over the last few decades. Heavy metals have also been linked to mental health issues like anger and depression. Even environmental toxins are causing more weight gain and obesity due to disrupting the endocrine system.

After my second baby, when my health was failing, I remember I started feeling really nauseous. Elsie was 3-months old at the time, and I did a million (slight exaggeration!) pregnancy tests, thinking the nausea was morning sickness. I went into panic mode: how could I cope having another baby when I felt so physically and mentally burned! It turned out I wasn't pregnant. Instead, my body was in such a state of burnout, that I had become ultra sensitive to chemicals in our home. The nausea was triggered by fake candles. And I also started experiencing heart palpitations, headaches and eye irritation, when using cleaning products. Even electromagnetic fields (EMF's) started triggering chest tightness and tingles in my arms. I eventually put two and two together. I was shocked at how physically ill I was feeling from the candles, cleaning products and electrical devices, and wondered what else they were doing to my insides. I did a major clean out of all the toxic candles, cleaning and skincare products, and swapped them out for natural products, essential oils, and my own DIY creations. I also invested in EMF protecting equipment. All my chemical-related symptoms disappeared immediately once my environment was cleaned up, and I became an advocate for living low tox, starting my first natural health business, Happy Biome - www.happybiome.com.au - a natural skincare and cleaning range, and educational DIY workshops.

Now I know it might feel a bit doom-and-gloom all this talk about a toxic world. But I promise you. Making some simple swaps and cleaning up your own environment - your home - can make a huge difference to your health, and to the planet. After reading this chapter, you'll know exactly where to look for toxins in your food, skincare and cleaning products, and how to swap them out for natural alternatives. You'll also learn about the toxic-burden of dirty electricity (EMF's) and mould, and how to protect yourself from these harmful toxins.

Toxins in food, skincare, beauty and cleaning products - Isla's story

Isla's body was toxic. We saw it on her labs. Her glutathione stores (important for detoxification) were burned-up, she was struggling to make bile, her oestrogen levels were through the roof, and her serotonin levels depleted. Added to that were toxic related symptoms, like hormonal issues, weight gain, insomnia and anxiety. Isla was surrounded by chemicals all day at her hair salon. Plus she loaded her face and body with department store makeup and products. And while she ate "clean" on her "healthy" days, the wine, the chocolate, and the processed foods, were only increasing her already high toxic load. Isla needed a major toxin overhaul.

In the 1970s, more than 87,000 chemicals were approved for commercial use. However only around 1,000 were tested for carcinogenic effects. And of those tested, 500 were deemed carcinogenic. This is mind-blowing, and pure negligence! Potentially *half* of the 87,000 chemicals in use in commercial products, could be making us very sick. Additionally, of the chemicals tested now, toxic labelling is required if only 50% or more of the animals tested with the chemical die. That's just madness. So if only 49% of animals die, then the chemical would be deemed fit for human consumption? And what of the surviving animals? Were they ever followed up long-term to assess for metabolic diseases, endocrine disruption or cancer? No.

These toxic products creep into your home and workspace so stealthily. They can hide in your food, your water, your skincare, cleaning and beauty products. They can sneak in through furniture, paint, candles, air fresheners and craft materials. One small exposure to a product might not do too much harm, but add up all the hidden chemicals in your home, and you can see how it could impact your body. While it's hard to completely strip your home bare of everything toxic, in this section I want to show you how to identify and remove the easy things, to make a dramatic impact.

First you have to get ingredient savvy. There are literally thousands of toxic chemicals you should ditch or stay away from, but here's a helpful list of the top 20 toxic chemicals found in skincare, cleaning, beauty and hygiene products:

TOP 20 TOXINS IN SKINCARE & CLEANING

- Chlorine/bleach
- Sodium lauryl sulphate
- Fragrance
- Formaldehyde
- Quarternium-15
- Ammonia
- Triclosan
- Phthalates
- Phenol
- 2-Butoxyethanol
- Flouride
- Microbeads
- Aluminium
- Parabens
- TEA & DEA
- Oxybenzone
- Retinyl Palmitate (Vitamin A palmitate)
- Propylene Glycol
- BHA
- Mineral Oil (petroleum jelly)

And here's a list of the top 20 nasty chemicals (artificial flavourings, additives and preservatives, and "natural" chemicals that can be harmful if consumed) found in food & drinks:

TOP 20 TOXINS IN FOOD & DRINKS

- Monosodium Glutumate (MSG)
- Artificial Food Colouring (Blue 1 & 2, Red 2, 3 & 40, Yellow 5 & 6, Green 3)
- Sodium Nitrate
- High-Fructose Corn Syrup
- Artificial Sweeteners (aspartame, sucralose, saccharin and acesulfame potassium)
- Carrageenan
- Sodium Benzoate
- Trans Fat / Partially hydrogenated oil
- Artificial Flavouring
- BHA/BHT
- Pesticides
- Sodium Sulfite
- Sulfur Dioxide
- Potassium Bromate
- Propyl Galate
- Butane
- Paraben
- Aluminium
- Chlorine
- Flouride

Let's have a look at a couple of these toxic chemicals - mineral oil and parabens - so you can understand where they might be hiding, and what they can do to the body.

Mineral oil is also know as petroleum jelly. Any Vaseline fans out there? Yep Vaseline is made out of petroleum jelly. Did you know it comes from the same place as gasoline? Gross! It's marketed as giving a hit of "moisture" in skincare products, but really, it does nothing to nurture, heal or restore. It slows cellular regeneration, which can damage collagen, elastin and connective tissue. It also forms a seal over the skin, which disrupts the body's ability to eliminate toxins. It has been linked to allergies, impaired brain function and can lead to birth defects. This last one horrifies me, as I was addicted to Vaseline from the time I was 10 years old to 28 years old, and when I was pregnant with my first baby, I smeared it all over my belly, to prevent stretch marks. I could've literally done damage to my unborn baby! Mineral oil is also a probable carcinogenic, and has been banned in the use of cosmetics in some countries.

Then there are parabens. It's commonly used as a preservative in skincare and cleaning products - *and* in food. It has hormone disrupting effects linked with cancer and shifts in natural puberty patterns. Scientists dispute the dangers saying that parabens, although rapidly absorbed through the skin, are excreted. However, a British Study at the University of Reading on 20 different samples of human breast tumours showed each sample had traces of parabens. The researchers concluded: "the detection in human breast tumours is of concern since parabens have been shown to mimic the action of the female hormone estrogen." Ummm, get lost parabens. I'd like to keep my breasts in tact thank you!

How to ditch the nasty chemicals
If you've ditched the processed foods and are eating more whole foods, as outlined in Chapter 7, you should have already ditched the nasty additives in foods and drinks, or at least dramatically reduced them. If you're still eating packaged foods, make sure you cross-check the ingredients list, to ensure there aren't any nasties sneaking in. And town-water should always be filtered, to clear out chlorine, fluoride and other harmful chemicals.

In regards to your skincare, beauty, cleaning and hygiene products, start getting label-savvy, and check out the ingredients in the products you are using. The list can be very long, especially if you're using toxic products. It will take some time to work through each product, but once you've discovered what's clean and what's not, and you find a replacement for the product, you won't have to think about it any longer. I've saved you the hassle of researching, with my Happy Biome skincare and cleaning product range - www.happybiome.com.au You can also download a DIY Skincare recipe book from my book's website - www.chrisandfilly.fm/book

Isla was feeling overwhelmed by this huge learning curve. After looking at the amount of products she was using, I knew reading through every ingredient would feel like running a never-ending marathon.

"I have a handy tool for you," I said to Isla. "It's going to make things so much quicker!"

I showed Isla the Think Dirty app. This is a handy little app that scans the barcodes of your personal care and beauty products, and immediately tells you if the product is "clean" or "dirty."

"Just make sure you type in Think Dirty *app* when searching in Google," I said to Isla with a little smile. "Because Think Dirty without the 'app' might take you somewhere completely different!"

Some other handy resources that I love to use to determine if a food, cosmetic or cleaning product is clean or dirty is the book *The Chemical Maze* by Bill Statham & Lindy Schneider, and their accompanying app. And the website www.ewg.org

Isla slowly worked through her products at home, and replaced them with natural alternatives from her local health food store. She even got into DIY-ing her own mineral makeup, after I taught her how easy (and cheap!) it is to make your own products, even your own professional-grade makeup. And as for her hair salon. She wasn't willing to quit her business. But she changed her hair products and dyes to more organic options, and ditched the commercial-grade cleaning products for natural ones.

EMF's – Hazel's story

Hazel was on technology all day long. She was constantly on the computer working. She always had AirPods plugged to her ears, constantly making phone calls. Her mobile phone lived in her pocket. The accumulation of EMF's were no doubt stressing out her adrenal glands, and adding more inflammation to her gut. But Hazel also had some other weird symptoms going on.

"My arms feel very painful to touch. Like they're on fire," Hazel explained. "And I've been getting ringing in the ears, almost daily."

"What about headaches?" I asked.

"Yes! Not everyday. They're coming and going. I can't pinpoint what's triggering them."

It turned out Hazel had started to develop an EMF sensitivity. This isn't uncommon with body system burnout. And while body system burnout can lead to EMF sensitivity, overexpose of EMF's can also cause body systems to breakdown. EMF sensitivity symptoms can be very random and varied. Common symptoms include insomnia, fatigue, dizziness, nerve pain, pins and needles, tinnitus, brain fog, gut issues, headaches. The list can go on!

EMF's emit from power lines, power boxes, electrical circuits in your walls, electrical appliances, WIFI, Xbox, phones and 4G/5G. It is caused by interruptions in the flow of normal 60-Hertz AC (alternating current) power traveling through wires and electrical systems in homes and other buildings. These interruptions result in voltage spikes, or surges, as well as frequency variations that combine to form a complex and potentially harmful electromagnetic field. The unused EMF's float around in your environment, and your own body sucks them up, which then disrupts your own electromagnetic circuits. There has been an exponential increase in the use of electronic devices over the past few decades, and data shows that EMF's can cause an abnormal stress response in the body, which breaks cells and DNA strands. Excessive EMF exposure has also been linked to the increasing rise of cancer, reproductive issues and neurobehavioral abnormalities.

Hazel's mouth dropped when I explained how taxing EMF's can be on the body. "So what are you saying?" Hazel said. "That I have to stop using my computer and mobile? How would I even be able to work!"

"Well, you could go live off-grid on top of the mountain," I joked.

"Not likely," Hazel said, with a humph.

Unless you're keen to live without technology, there are other ways you can protect yourself from harmful EMF's, while still being able to work and live with technology. Here are some things we helped Hazel integrate into her life:

- Hazel unplugged all electronics, like WIFI, the TV and the kids' Xbox, before going to bed.
- She kept her mobile phone in aeroplane mode while not in use, and ditched the blue-tooth AirPods. When she needed to use earphones, she used the wired earphones, as these cut-off the excessive EMF's that blue-tooth earphones bring.
- She set up her workspace with EMF protective devices, including a laptop shield, radiation blanket and blue shield plugins that drew dirty electricity from circuits.
- Hazel prioritised getting outside on her lunch breaks, and taking her shoes off and walking or sitting barefoot on the grass. This is called "earthing" and has been shown to discharge EMF's from your body.
- If feeling very "charged," Hazel would also do an epsom salt bath at night, to release excess energy.

Dr Kristy Goodwin in her book *Dear Digital*, also has some fantastic micro-habits that are easy to implement, to help reduce technology time and to disconnect so that the brain and body can recovery from technology use. I highly recommend reading her book.

Mould – Rose's story

Rose lived in an old farm cottage. It was perfect in every way. High ceilings, the quaintest kitchen. It was on a beautiful five acre block. Surrounded by trees and a bubbling river. But the things was, Rose's house was also harbouring hidden black mould.

Exposure to toxic moulds from water damaged buildings is very common and completely under-diagnosed. In fact, at least 50% of homes and 60% of commercial buildings have water damage. While some people can live with mould without major issues, it is estimated that 25% of the population have a genetic mutation of the HLA-DR gene, which makes them more susceptible to mould toxicity. That's right - a quarter of the population could be experiencing body burnout symptoms due to mould sensitivity. Plus, chuck in other body system imbalances, and a dysregulated nervous system from psychological stress, and it can become a recipe for mould disaster. Mould produces allergens, irritants and toxic substances, or spores, that float around in your environment, and get inhaled into your lungs. The spores can then reproduce in your system, and take camp in your fat cells, causing all sorts of symptoms like allergies, respiratory infections, fatigue, brain fog, muscle and joint pain, gut issues, and multiple chemical sensitivity.

I started suspecting mould sensitivity in Rose when her symptom improvements were inconsistent. Some months she was doing good, and then other months, out of nowhere, her fatigue, brain fog, thrush and low mood would flare up again. This is a common pattern in patients with mould sensitivity, especially if they are still living in a mouldy environment. Rose also reported ringing in the ears, and a constant sniffle, cough and itchy eyes, especially in the wintertime - all classic symptoms of mould sensitivity.

"Rose, you live in a pretty old house, and it gets very damp in wintertime. I think you need to start looking for sources of mould in your home," I said.

"I'm pretty sure there's no mould in our house," Rose said. "I mean, sometimes the windowsills get a bit mouldy in the wintertime, but I keep it clean."

"The thing is, Rose, mould is often hidden."

Where to find mould in your home

Mould loves water, moisture, humid air, and dark, warm places. Here are common places you might find mould:

- Bathroom
- Laundry (including inside the washing machine seals on front-loader doors)
- Kitchen (including inside appliances)
- Leaky roof
- Windowsills (condensation)
- Food
- Rubbish bins
- Diffusers
- Ice-maker in fridge
- Air conditioners (also in cars!)
- Water filters
- Chipboard (can easily breed mould)
- Dusty areas (dust feeds mould when moisture is added)
- Kids bathtub toys
- CPAP machines for sleep apnea
- Furniture
- Bedding
- Pot plants
- Inside walls and under floors

Rose and her husband did a thorough investigation of their house using an environmental mould company. Sure enough, they found black mould in some walls and skirting boards. As well as in pot plants, and their heat pump.

To test my theory about mould sensitivity, I asked Rose to go sleep in her newly built massage studio on her property, and try to spend the least amount of time in her home. When she did this, she felt an improvement in her symptoms.

When we caught up for a follow-up consult after the trial, Rose said: "To tell you the truth, I always feel better when we go on holidays. I thought that was because I was less 'stressed' but maybe it's actually because of the mould?"

"I think it is!" I said, slapping my hand on the table. There's nothing quite like further connecting the dots.

We confirmed my suspicion with a mould allergy lab test from Nutripath (check out Appendix for more info) which showed Rose was reacting to mould in her environment.

How to get rid of mould

Rose needed to get rid of the mould – and pronto! – so she could fully heal her body systems. You see, the more mould attacks your system, the more it damages your mitochondria, neurotransmitters and detoxification nutrients – all things Rose was trying to restore. In addition, a mould issue can feed a candida overgrowth, making it really hard to rebalance the gut and vaginal ecosystem. Luckily Rose and her husband had an investment property they could move into, while they renovated their farm cottage to get rid of the mould.

If you also have a mould problem in your home, here's what you can do:

- **Chuck it!** Anything that can be chucked away, chuck it. Especially if you can't clean the mould off it effectively. Ditch those mouldy bathtub toys, pillows, plants, etc.
- **Clean it!** Anything that can be easily cleaned, clean it. Using a natural DIY mould cleaner recipe (like water, witch hazel and essential oils) is best. 8% hydrogen peroxide can also be effective against mould. Don't use toxic mould killers as they rarely kill mould spores, and can cause mould resistance.
- **Prevention!** Mould thrives in moist, humid areas and eats dust. Regularly vacuum dust (always empty the bag outside), wipe down moisture (from windows, windowsills, bench tops), and purify your air (either with opened windows or with an air purifier).
- **Repair/Renovate!** If you have water damage in your home, get in touch with a builder and repair the wet/mouldy areas where needed.
- **Relocate!** If your mouldy home is beyond help – relocate! I know this isn't going to be achievable for most people in a month. But you could think about making this part of your

future goals. If you are looking to buy or rent a new home, look for any water damage or signs of mould, and only move in if it's mould-free.

When Rose removed herself from a mouldy environment, she finally responded consistently to our body systems treatments. And as her gut health and detox pathways improved, and as she worked on her self-limiting beliefs which helped to regulate her nervous system and body into a place of safety, and implemented better sleeping and eating habits, she became more resilient to mould, even though she had genetic mutations making her more susceptible. And that, dear reader, is the beauty of holistic healing and functional medicine.

Now that your home is clean of nasty toxins, it's time to move to the last chapter of this book: how to create a happy home, supportive of your health, happiness and that of your family.

SUMMARY
LOW TOX HOME

As a summary, here's what you need to do to create a toxin-free home and space conducive for healing:

- Identify any hidden nasty chemicals in packaged foods and drinks, and in cleaning, skincare, beauty and hygiene products. Toss them out and replace them with natural alternatives.
- Reduce EMF exposure in your home and workspace by turning off technology and appliances when not using them, and by implementing EMF protective equipment. Get outside and "earth" as well.
- Identify any hidden sources of mould in your home, and toss it, clean it, renovate it, or move away from it completely.

CHAPTER 12

Happy Home

Introduction
In this chapter, you'll learn all about the importance of creating a happy home, especially within the scope of ending your body burnout, and having vibrant health and happiness for life.

    I'm sure you would agree with me, that as a busy, juggling woman, a huge stressor in your life is likely your relationships. If there's constant bickering between you and your partner, if your kids are triggering you with their whining or neediness or snappy-teenage remarks, if you feel like you're doing everything for your family, and your tank is running empty, or if you're experiencing abuse, all of these things are going to add extra stress to your already overflowing stress bucket. Stress equals body system burnout, remember. In order to truly break free from energy, mood and gut issues, your relationships are going to have to be inspected.

In addition, family and close friends or work colleagues can either make or break your healing journey. There's plenty of research that links success in health to a supportive network. If your whole family and those who are close to you are behind you, cheering you on, even making healthy changes alongside you, your chance of success will skyrocket. However, if there's constant resistance from your family, if they are sabotaging your good intentions, or if they are downright putting you down for your desire for personal transformation, you are more likely to fall off track at some point.

After reading this chapter, you'll have a deeper understanding of why it is important to create a loving relationship with yourself first, before you can improve relationships with others. You'll also discover how you can step into your power and become a leader for change, aligning your family with your own ending body burnout mission. At the end of the day, you probably started this journey, not just to resolve your health issues, but to also become more connected to those you love the most. Humans crave connection. We're hardwired this way. This chapter is the ultimate prize of what you can gain, when you holistically end your body burnout, once and for all.

Healthy relationships start with yourself

I've spoken extensively throughout this book about how important it is to have a healthy relationship with yourself. Without this, it's not only impossible to fully and deeply heal, but also very difficult to have deep and connected relationships with others. Having a healthy relationship with yourself is crucial, if you ever want to overcome getting "triggered" constantly by others, so that you can achieve healthy, happy relationships with those you love. If you think otherwise, you're lying to yourself. Period. You might think that you're a better mum or parter or sister or friend or boss if you put others first. But by doing this, you're betraying your own relationship with yourself. Betrayal is always attached with guilt, shame and hatred. If you feel self-guilt, shame or hatred, how can you ever know how to have a thriving relationship with others? Even worse is lying to yourself, and pretending like you don't have any self-love issues.

Let's see how an insecure relationship with self shows up negatively in relationships in Rose, Hazel and Isla:

Rose
Rose's deepest self-limiting belief and fear that she was unlovable wasn't just affecting her health. It was also causing major issues in her relationships. Because her internal love-dial was low, she was constantly seeking love and acceptance externally, from others. This made her needy for love, a people pleaser. She was constantly doing everything else for her family, not from a noble desire to be a loving mother and wife and therapist (as she had originally thought), but from a deep fear that if she didn't, she would not receive any love, and thus her deepest fear of being unlovable would be confirmed. This of course led to her body burnout, but she also became resentful towards her family - *they* were the ones making her exhausted. Because she hid behind "doing for others," and because she feared rejection, she also failed to communicate effectively. Her family had no idea how she felt, or that she even desperately needed help.

Hazel
Hazel, deep down, didn't believe she was "enough," just as she was. Although she wasn't aware consciously of this fact when we first met, her behaviours showed she was consumed by inadequacy. And this limiting self-belief spurred her addictive doing behaviour, to the point of body burnout. It was also hugely affecting her relationship with her kids. She believed she was showing "love" to her children by being the bread-winner, and bringing financial security to her family - something *their Dad* never did. However, deep-down, she had created her overworking patterns as a way of excusing herself from emotionally loving the kids, because deep-down she believed she didn't have what it takes to be a good Mum. It was obvious she wasn't cut out to be a "good wife"

(that was validated when her husband left her). So it was only a matter of time before the kids left too, right? Getting "stuck" in work, was a behavioural pattern that worked perfectly to get out of showing up as an exceptional mum. If she screwed up the kids, or they ended up hating her, it was the work that did it, not her "true self." Her children's love cups, of course, weren't getting filled (the Nanny couldn't do this in place of Hazel), and this showed up in their ratty behaviour, competing for Mum's attention, fighting and squabbling until Hazel reared her "Dragon Mum's" angry head up and - snapped!

Isla
Isla deemed herself unworthy. This stemmed from the stories she created about herself to make sense of her childhood trauma, as well as her inability to have children in the past. It was hugely affecting her body systems and the decisions she made around her health. It also carried with it self-shame. Isla was wounded inside, and she was constantly trying to project a different "version" of herself - the spunky bright hairdresser, the life of the party - in an attempt to protect herself from not being "found out" about her worthlessness, and out of a desperate desire to be loved. The problem was, she was so scared of being rejected, that she rarely stood up for herself in her relationships. When her girlfriends brought in the bubbles after work, she drank it alongside of them, so that she didn't "offend" them. When her partner (who had his own baggage) treated her poorly, she let him, because she didn't feel like she was worthy of being treated the way she desired. And even though sex boiled up somatic tension in her body from past trauma, she feigned indifference to her body, and went along with her partner's sexual advances, for fear of rejection. All the while she felt like an empty shell.

As you can see a dysfunctional relationship with yourself will only end up in frustrated and broken relationships, and additional stress for yourself. For a deeper look into personal insecurity and how this can sabotage relationships, there is no better book than *Leverage* by Jaemin Frazer.

Mission aligned

Once you've created a loving and secure relationship with yourself, and you're super clear about your vision of who you want to be, and your mission to end your own body burnout, it's time to get your family and those close to you aligned with your mission.

You want my family to change as well? Are you kidding!

You might think I'm being idealistic here. I get it. I know getting the family onboard can feel like moving a big fat stubborn elephant. So let's be realistic first. If you try to rush in and get your family making healthy changes *before* you change yourself, it's going to be mission impossible. Without increasing your own capacity with new empowering beliefs, better health and energy so you can do the work required, as well as having the resources to show your family how to make change, you'll lose steam and give up quickly. So first, make a commitment to yourself to get *your self* sorted first, and be ok to let go of "mummy-guilt" that you're eating or living healthier than the kids (it's only for the short term). Then, make sure your family are aware and ready to support you in *your* personal mission. You're not asking them to have a transformation for themselves (at least not yet), you're simply asking them to support you with whatever you need to heal from body burnout. That might look like helping around a bit more with the housework, so you don't have to do so much. Or to eat their junk food away from the house, to eliminate temptations for yourself. Or to get your partner to go to another room to watch Netflix on their phone, so you can go to sleep without distraction. This might feel completely unnatural or out of your comfort zone. But as you start to recreate new stories about yourself - you are loveable, you are strong, you are worthy, you are a success - then you will begin to expect nothing less. Because ultimately, as Jaemin Frazer says in *Leverage*, you are the prize, and in order to win and keep the prize, others must treat you the way you deserve.

Chris, my partner in marriage and business, always says, "what you allow, you encourage." This is a maxim Chris often uses with clients during coaching sessions. It's also something he has said to me, many times. I remember filling out a Census form a couple of years ago. Going into completing the form, I was already feeling frustrated and a bit burned-out, doing all the housework and cleaning, with little help from my family. I would suppress my frustration for days, sometimes even weeks, resentfully doing the chores, until it would reach a tipping point and I would snap: "Why doesn't anyone clean up around here? You're all a bunch of pigs!" My boiler really hit exploding point when I filled in the Census and clearly saw that Chris and I were working the same amount of hours, yet he was only doing an hour or two of housework a week, while I was doing 20+ hours! Um, recipe for working mum burnout! I stormed down to Chris's office, then and there, my chest puffed out, and jabbed the Census form in front of his face. Without any judgement, he simply said: "Filly, what you allow, you encourage." I felt the urge to slap him. But I adulted-up, took a big breath, sat down, and talked about the issue.

Turns out I wasn't allowing others to help out. I wasn't teaching them how. I was expecting them to use initiative (or read my mind!) and just "do" it. And I didn't even give them time to do the chores, because I kept rushing in to do them first. There was no clear expectation of who was in charge of what. My family expected me to do it all, because that's what I'd been unconsciously encouraging all along! Upon further analysis, this behaviour was modelled by my mother, and her mother before that. It's generational, and steeped in patriarchy. And also extremely common in modern working mums today (a study looking at 20,000 households found that after the first child is born, women do far more housework than men, and that, as the children grow up, the dynamic only worsens). It could've been easy to point fingers at my parents or a patriarchal society for making me this way, but after doing my own personal development work I realised my behaviour stemmed from the old dysfunctional beliefs I created about myself as a child: I needed to prove I was "capable" of looking after the household, and when I did, others would approve of me, and most especially my mother. The crazy thing was, it had nothing to do with disapproval from my mum or anyone else. But rather the idea I created about myself as a kid, that I was somehow weak and incapable, which carried out into adulthood. Because my actions were driven from a place of fear and the need to prove myself, asking for help from my family wouldn't work, because they couldn't do the job "well enough," and that would be a direct reflection on me. And so my behaviour ended up being quite controlling, and not allowing others a chance to help. Madness, right?

The point of the story is: what you allow, you encourage. If you continue living out your self-limiting beliefs, if you continue doing everything for everyone else, if you continue letting others treat you poorly, if you continue over-doing and being controlling, you will not only remain in body burnout, but you'll never experience deep and loving relationships, which will only cause more stress to your already overtaxed system.

So stand up, be a leader, and align your family with your mission. Start encouraging something new. Here's some steps to get started:

- First, get really clear and honest with yourself: what are you allowing to happen, that you don't like? What are you constantly doing - or not doing - that saps your soul, and causes body burnout? Are you doing anything out of resentment, drudgery or even downright hatred?
- Next, get clear on what you'd like to delegate to other family members, or to hired help.
- Also get clear on what you need emotionally from your family. What do you need from your partner? What do you need from your children?
- Get clear on what support you need from your family, to make healing possible. What are they currently doing that might sabotage your good intentions, or that are quite literally making you sick?
- Schedule a time to discuss your expectations with your family. Enter this discussion as a leader, not as a victim or out of spite or neediness. Clearly pitch what you desire, and allow space for negotiation so that it is a win/win for everyone.
- Finish the discussion off by writing up a family contract, outlining expectations for all family members. Make this a fun, family activity and get everyone to sign it at the end.
- Regularly review the contract as a whole family, and amend as needed.

The faster your family can become aligned with what you're trying to achieve, the faster they will move up to your level.

Become the leader - Isla's story

You might've tried to get your family onboard already. If they got onboard right away - great! You have a rare family unit. More than likely, however, your first attempts were fruitless. The kids probably rolled their eyes at you, and kept playing their video games. Or your partner took it personally, and you ended up having a fight. If this was the case, you were probably stuck somewhere in the Drama Triangle.

Stephen Karpman's Drama Triangle (which we have adapted) explains why you might be struggling to instigate change in your family. The model looks at how dysfunctional relationships play out by looking at the stories we tell ourselves and how we show up in relationships (as shown in figure 12.1):

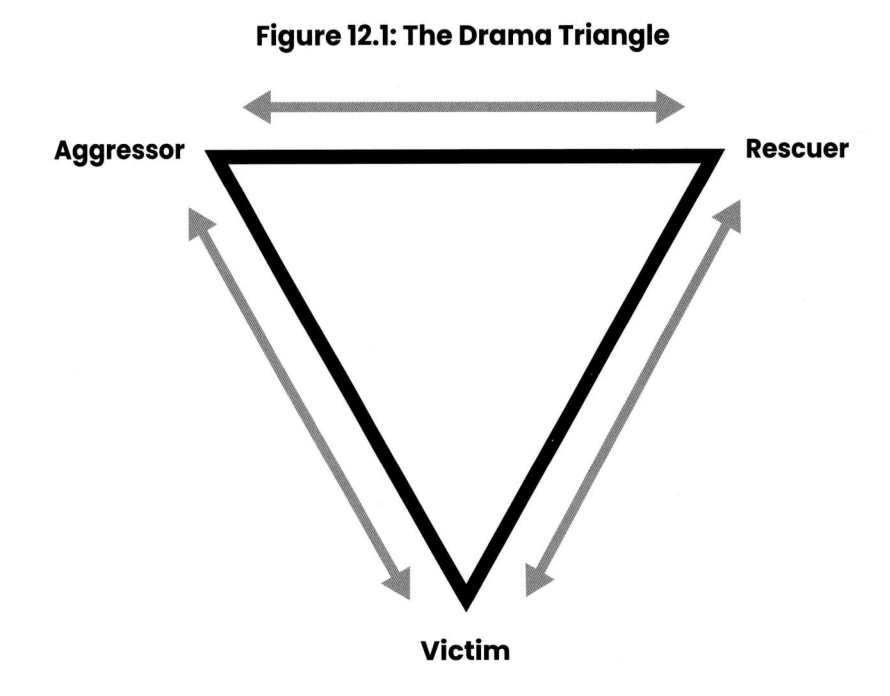

Figure 12.1: The Drama Triangle

Aggressor ↔ **Rescuer**

Victim

The Aggressor

The aggressor plays the role of the bully. They come across as aggressive, demanding, spiteful and scornful - either openly or passively. They are quick to point the finger at the victim, and are not open to seeing other people's views. Mama, are you playing the role of the aggressor when you're trying to get your family on board with your mission? Are you coming across as judgey, controlling and critical? *It's my way, or the highway!* If so, you will always be met with resistance and resentment by those you are trying to control.

The Victim

The victim's position is "poor me!" They are helpless, needy, fretful, and often complain about their "lot" in life. They blame others - or situations - for their dire circumstances, and defer to others to fix them/their issues. Are you coming to the table as a victim, when trying to make change within your family? Are you blaming them - or their behaviour - for your body burnout? Are you trying to get them to change by nagging and being needy? If you're behaving like a victim, you'll never instigate change, as you'll always be expecting someone else (a rescuer) to wave a magic wand and fix it all, or you'll continue to lay blame on someone or something.

The Rescuer

The rescuer exists to rescue victims. While it sounds noble and compassionate on the surface, underneath a rescuer doesn't actually value other people's capacity to help themselves. They like to be needed, so they will continue to hold a victim captive, never quite allowing them to grow and evolve. Rescuers are prone to meddling unnecessarily, and can come across as engulfing. By focusing their energy on "fixing" the victim, they draw away from working on their own dysfunctions. Are you coming into your family discussions as the rescuer, the hero? Saving your family from disease and dysfunction? Shoving your own beliefs and wants onto them? And not really looking deep into your own dysfunctions? If so, your family will see right through you.

Break free from the Drama Triangle

Can you see yourself in the Drama Triangle? You might be acting out one predominant role, or you might be pinging around all three, depending on how others respond to you.

To get out of aggressor, victim or rescuer mode, you need to become a leader. You need to see change. Be the change. Lead the change. Not out of force, or neediness, or from a place of hypocrisy. A leader focuses on outcomes, rather than problems. She leads from a place of wisdom. She has walked the walk, not just talked the talk. A leader empowers and coaches others to work through their own problems, without trying to solve it for them. A leader challenges others – not in a critical way, but in a way that holds others accountable, and leads to growth. When you become a leader in your own family, your family will want to follow you. This is the ultimate prize: you don't just get yourself healthy, but you also create health and happiness in your family.

Isla was not sure about this. She'd hidden from confrontation all her life, out of a desperate neediness to be loved. She was so scared to tell her partner to stop pouring wine in her glass at night, in case she offended him, or her worst fear – he threatened to leave her. And she was extremely skeptical that he would change the way he was eating. Before Isla even attempted the conversation with her partner, we helped her first heal her broken relationship with herself. This enabled Isla to step into her power, and out of the role of victim. She created a new vision for herself, created steps to become that new woman, and began creating that new woman. She then made a time for a meeting with her partner, where she set out her expectations, clearly. During our next online group coaching session, Chris asked: "How did that go for you?" Isla was excited to report that she had had the meeting as planned. Her partner was not offended about her request to stop pouring her wine. But she was a bit disappointed because he continued to drink the wine at night, and continued eating their old regular meals, while she ate her "healthy" meal and drank her glass of kombucha beside him.

"I don't know how long I can last like this?" Isla said, I could see in her eyes that she was beginning to doubt herself again.

"Remember Isla," Chris said. "See the change. Be the change. Lead the change."

A month later, during a group session, Isla's eyes lit up when we started the session with wins. "I don't know how," Isla said. "But just this past week my husband announced that he's going to give up alcohol for this whole month! And he's actually wanting to eat the same food I am."

"You know exactly how," Chris said. "See the change. Be the change. Lead the change."

I hope this chapter has helped sum up our ending body burnout method and the beautiful, ripple-effect that occurs when you do. I have a big vision, bigger than just our functional medicine practice. I see a world where women can make a huge impact in this world, without burning-out. At the end of the day, our method, encapsulated in this book, empowers women to be their own healer, by teaching them how. And that's going to have far-reaching effects on their family, their community, and the world.

Change one woman, and we change the world.

Change one woman, and we change generations.

Beauty, I'm so excited to see you shine!

SUMMARY
HAPPY HOME

As a summary, here's what you need to do to get your family on board with your healing journey, and as a natural flow-on effect, achieve a happier home:

- First and foremost, heal your own relationship with yourself.
- Get your family aligned with your personal mission to end your body burnout, and create clear expectations for what you need in order to heal.
- Become a leader in your family, to instigate change, not just in yourself, but also in your loved ones.

Conclusion

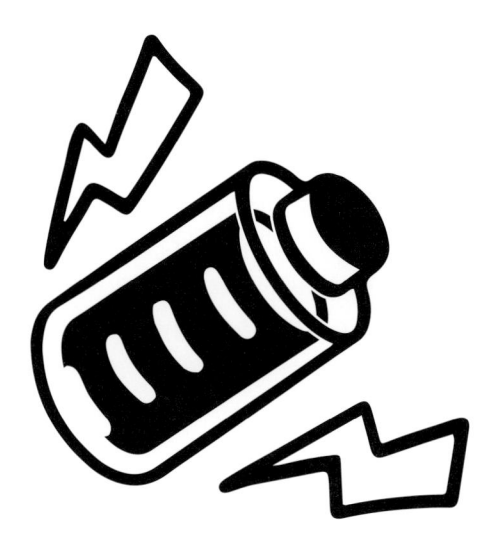

So there you have it, busy lady juggling all the things! The four-step process to ending your body burnout, once and for all. As you learned, the first step is to get answers, a clear diagnosis of what body systems have burned out, which have then led to your energy, mood and gut issues. Once you know what body systems are imbalanced, you then need to identify *why* these systems have broken down in the first place - what are the root-causes, and most importantly, what is your deepest root-cause driving all other causes? The following three steps, as you learned in this book, help you to identify the mind, body and environment root-causes, and what you need to do to address them. If you haven't done our

Ending Body Burnout Assessment yet, now is the time to pinpoint where your body burnout and root-causes lie - http://chrisandfilly.fm/scorecard

Scan to do scorecard

When you address your body burnout at a deep and holistic level outlined in this book, when you go beyond just supplements and diet and meditation, you will finally *end* your body burnout. You'll no longer have to practitioner or doctor or course or diet hop, getting a little bit of relief here and there. You'll no longer have to experience your same old burnout issues flaring up, time and time again. Your results will last, for life, because you are now your own self-regulator and self-healer. Follow the steps outlined in this book and you'll have more energy, more productivity (without *doing more*), and a deep love for yourself and for those around you.

So, you have two options right now:

Option 1. Keep doing the same thing
After reading this book, it just all seems too hard. You don't know where to start. Maybe you've tried in the past to seek help, with little results. Maybe you're scared to invest your money into something that "might not work." Maybe changing feels like too much of a gamble. Maybe you don't have enough "time" or "energy" to do the deep work of healing. Maybe you're hoping for a "quick-fix" so you jump from practitioner to practitioner, or supplement to supplement, trying to get a quick solution. Maybe you don't value yourself enough to give yourself the space to heal. Maybe you don't believe you can heal. Maybe you think you are destined to stay exhausted and grumpy forever.

There are many stories we tell ourselves when we're faced with an opportunity to heal. Remember: these are just *stories*. All stories are fictitious (even what is thought to be "true" ones). Why? Because the storyteller (you) is speaking from a subjective point of view. Your lens is tainted by your current belief-system that you have about yourself.

If you continue to stay stuck in your unproductive stories, one of two things will happen:

A. Either you will keep doing the same thing and you will remain the same. You'll continue feeling overwhelmed and anxious. You'll continue to struggle to sleep. You'll continue to drag yourself throughout the day because you're so fatigued. You'll continue being plagued with heartburn or bloating or chronic pain. You'll continue to struggle with PMS or painful periods. You'll continue to be irritable and snappy towards your family. And you will continue to feel foggy at work.

B. Or, you will keep doing the same thing and…get worse! Suddenly you'll find yourself on a restricted diet because you're reacting to almost every food - even healthy ones. You'll have to drop down to two days a week of work (or give up your business or career completely!) because you're struggling to get through the day. You'll find your marriage at the edge of break-up because you're such a "monster" to be around. You'll start hating being around your kids because you're so exhausted and on the brink of falling apart; their energy and neediness irritate you.

Not a pretty picture, is it? If you are anything like how I used to be, it was these fears of not just my body falling apart (even more so!), but also my family, business and my life falling apart that pushed me towards change. I knew if I didn't do something, I would end up far worse than my already unhappy and chaotic state.

Option 2. Do something different

The second option: you could do something different, and get a different (and better) result. I know this may seem scary. I know you may feel like you've tried many times. But if you stay stuck in your current state of being, nothing will change - at least not for the better.

Chris and I have both been on our own healing journeys. We know what it feels like to be stressed-out and worn-out, and all the physical and emotional symptoms that come along with this state of being. We know what to do - *and* what it takes - to heal from body burnout. Not just from a practitioner point of view (of which we have spent half a million dollars on our education, with the world's best mentors, and have studied and practiced for over a combined 25+ years), but also from a very visceral and personal point of view. We were in the trenches too!

We were both led to our professions (our callings!) because of the need to heal ourselves. And, with the help of our many mentors, we have learned how to not only get to the root-cause, but also to end body burnout for good. It took us many years to get to where we are now. The good news? We can turn your decades into days (so to speak!). Instead of you, alone, trying many, many years to try to even figure out what the heck is wrong with you, we can accelerate this process with our proven ending body burnout method. Finally you can share the load of your issues, with someone who has been there and knows how to navigate the maze of body burnout.

So, what story are you going to tell yourself? What path are you going to choose?

If nothing changes, nothing changes.

And just know: the deeper your body falls apart, the deeper your root-causes become entrenched, the longer and harder it will be to turn things around.

There is never a better time than now, beautiful lady. You, my dear, who is so worthy of shining!

And in case you were wondering...
Rose
Rose did recover from her body burnout. Her physical healing really skyrocketed once we worked out the mould issue, which allowed her body to respond to the therapeutic protocols to restore her brain, mitochondria and gut health. Supporting her methylation pathways, longer-term, also meant she could function optimally, despite her genetic mutations. She was back to exercising (mindfully, mind you!) again. She had more stamina in her massage therapy practice. And she still had energy after work to spend time with her family, rather than flaking out on the couch.

The real "magic pill" for Rose, though, was learning to love herself, first and foremost. This self-acceptance allowed her to break through the motherhood martyrdom pattern that fed her body burnout in the first place. She no longer needed love from others to feel like she was enough, because her own internal love-cup was filled. And this finally allowed her to give herself permission to honour herself, and to put her self first.

Isla
Isla also overcame body burnout and rebalanced her hormones, brain, gut and detox pathways. She finally felt the calmest she had ever felt in her life, and even her weight shifted (while doing *less* intense exercise!). Environmental chemicals were really burning out her systems, and when she was able to change up the way she ran her hair salon, what she used in the home *and* reduced the wine and bubbles and decadent foods, her body systems were finally able to heal.

For this to become possible, Isla needed to believe herself worthy of healing. Otherwise she would've continued, forever, yo-yoing from one health-kick to another. Wasting yet another round of money, time, and sanity. It required reframing her self-limiting beliefs. She was good, she was worthy, she was enough, just as she was. And it also required doing unconscious trauma release work, to bring her system back to safety. This allowed her to make transformational lifestyle and behavioural shifts, and not just in herself, but also in her family. This was the secret sauce that made ending body burnout possible.

Hazel
Hazel experienced some good wins while working with us. As challenging as it was, she got through the elemental diet and cleared her SIBO. Her gut issues improved dramatically - no bloating, and bowel movements were more regulated. She also implemented some self-care into her busy life, to help reduce stress and support her adrenals. She created a more structured and sleep-promoting evening routine. She switched off from work more, and spent time with her kids.

She did become aware of where her addictive-doing patterns stemmed from - a need to prove that she was "good enough." Hazel, however, didn't complete her full program. She ejected when work got "too busy," stuck again in her addictive-doing patterns. Awareness was not enough for Hazel to make the complete transformation needed to *end* her body burnout. I later found out that Hazel's gut issues flared up again, and she was learning to "live with it."

References

Introduction
'Facts & Figures about Mental Health,' *Black Dog Institute*, https://www.blackdoginstitute.org.au/wp-content/uploads/2020/04/1-facts_figures.pdf

'Mental Health Link To Work Life Balance,' *Latrobe University*, 2015, https://www.latrobe.edu.au/news/articles/2015/release/mental-health-link-to-work-life-balance

'Mental Health Working Mums,' *Benenden Health*, https://www.benenden.co.uk/be-healthy/work/mental-health-working-mums/

W Tuohy, 'Two thirds of working parents 'struggle to care for their own health,' *The Sydney Morning Herald*, 2019, https://www.smh.com.au/lifestyle/life-and-relationships/two-thirds-of-working-parents-struggle-to-care-for-their-own-health-20191028-p534z9.html

L Corduff, 'The survey on women: sleep, stress, sex and more,' unpublished survey, data collected October 2022.

Step 1: The Body Systems
D Kalish, *Kalish Institute of Functional Medicine*, https://www.kalishinstitute.com/

Chapter 1: Neuroendocrine System
J Wilson, *Adrenal Fatigue: The 21st Century Stress Syndrome.* Smart Publications, 2001.

Nutripath Integrative and Pathology Services, www.nutripath.com.au

L Briden, *Hormone Repair Manual: Every woman's guide to healthy hormones after 40*. Pan MacMillan, 2021.

Chapter 2: Gastrointestinal System

M Gershon, *The Second Brain: A Groundbreaking New Understanding of Nervous Disorders of the Stomach and Intestine*. Harper Collins, 1999.

J Weinstock, 'Do We Need Worms to Promote Immune Health?' *Clin Rev Allergy Immunol*, vol. 49, no. 2, 2015, pp. 227-31, https://pubmed.ncbi.nlm.nih.gov/25326880/

M Gainza-Ciraqui et al., 'Production of carcinogenic acetaldehyde by Candida albicans from patients with potentially malignant oral mucosal disorders,' Journal of Oral Pathology Medicine, vol. 42, no. 3, pp. 243-9, https://pubmed.ncbi.nlm.nih.gov/22909057/

K Lynch, 'Hiatus Hernia,' *MSD Manual*, 2022, https://www.msdmanuals.com/en-au/professional/gastrointestinal-disorders/esophageal-and-swallowing-disorders/hiatus-hernia

N Lapid, 'How Villi Help With Digestion,' *Very Well Health*, 2023, https://www.verywellhealth.com/understanding-intestinal-villi-562555

P Kahrilas et al., 'Approaches to the Diagnosis and Grading of Hiatal Hernia,' *Best Practice Research Clinical Gastroenterology*, vol. 22, no. 4, pp. 601-616, 2008, https://www.ncbi.nlm.nih.gov/pmc/articles/PMC2548324/

J Bures et al., 'Small intestinal bacterial overgrowth syndrome,' *World Journal of Gastroenterology*, vol. 16, no. 24, pp. 2978-2990, 2010, https://www.ncbi.nlm.nih.gov/pmc/articles/PMC2890937/

A Bradford, 'How the Small Intestine Works,' *Live Science*, 2018, https://www.livescience.com/52048-small-intestine.html

Chapter 3: Detoxification System

A Stuart, *Low Tox Life: A Handbook for a Healthy You and a Happy Planet*. Murdoch Books, 2018.

B Lynch, *Dirty Genes: A Breakthrough Program to Treat the Root Cause of Illness and Optimize Your Health*. Harper Collins, 2020.

Chapter 4: Empowered Mind

J Frazer, *Unhindered: The 7 Essential Practices for Overcoming Insecurity*. Jaemin Frazer and Associates, 2020.

D Hawkins, *The Map of Consciousness Explained: A Proven Energy Scale to Actualize Your Ultimate Potential*. Hay House, 2020.

J Shaffer, 'Neuroplasticity and Clinical Practice: Building Brain Power for Health,' Front Psychology, vol. 7, no. 1118, 2016, https://www.ncbi.nlm.nih.gov/pmc/articles/PMC4960264/

L Hay, *Heal Your Body: The Mental Causes for Physical Illness and the Metaphysical Way to Overcome Them*. Hay House, 2004.

Chapter 5: Calm Mind

TS. Sathyanarayana Roa & V Indla, 'Work, family or personal life: Why not all three?,' *Indian Journal of Psychiatry*, vol. 52, no. 4, pp. 295-297, https://www.ncbi.nlm.nih.gov/pmc/articles/PMC3025152/

N LePera, *How To Do The Work: Recognise Your Patterns, Heal From Your Past + Create Your Self*. Hachette, 2021.

W Cole, *Gut Feelings: Healing the Shame-Fuelled Relationship Between What You Eat and How You Feel*. Yellow Kite, 2023.

P Chek, *How To Eat, Move & Be Healthy!*. C.H.E.K. Institute, 2001.

B Van Der Kolk, *The Body Keeps The Score: Mind, Brain and Body In Transformation of Trauma*. Penguin Press, 2014.

B Chapman, 'Emotion Suppression and Mortality Risk Over a 12-Year Follow-up,' *Journal of Psychosomatic Research*, vol. 75, no. 4, pp. 381-385, 2014, https://www.ncbi.nlm.nih.gov/pmc/articles/PMC3939772/

Chapter 6: Organised Mind

S Covey, *The 7 Habits of Highly Effective People: Powerful Lessons in Personal Change*. Simon & Schuster, 2011.

J Frazer, *Unhindered: The 7 Essential Practices for Overcoming Insecurity*. Jaemin Frazer and Associates, 2020.

Chapter 7: Restorative Nutrition

C Shanahan, *Deep Nutrition: Why Your Genes Need Traditional Food*. Flatiron Books, 2017.

Chapter 8: Restorative Sleep

P Check, *How To Eat, Move & Be Healthy!*. C.H.E.K. Institute, 2001.

L Geddes, *Chasing The Sun: The New Science of Sunlight and How it Shapes Our Bodies and Minds*. Wellcome Collection, 2019.

TS. Wiley, *Light's Out: Dying for a Good's Night Sleep? Sleep, Sugar and Survival*. Atria Books, 2001.

M Breus, *Good Night: The Sleep Doctor's 4-Week Program to Better Sleep and Better Health*. EP Dutton, 2006.

E Suni, 'How Much Sleep Do We Really Need?', *Sleep Foundation*, 2023, https://www.sleepfoundation.org/how-sleep-works/how-much-sleep-do-we-really-need

M Breus, *The Power of When: Learn the Best Time To Do Everything*. Ebury Digital, 2016.

K Goodwin, *Dear Digital, We Need To Talk: A Guilt-Free Guide To Taming Your Tech Habits and Thriving in a Distracted World*. Major Street Publishing, 2023.

Chapter 9: Restorative Movement

B Stubbs et al., 'Relationship between sedentary behavior and depression: A mediation analysis of influential factors across the lifespan among 42,469 people in low- and middle-income countries,' *Journal of Affective Disorders*, March 15, pp. 229-238, 2018, https://pubmed.ncbi.nlm.nih.gov/29329054/

J Park et al., 'Sedentary Lifestyle: Overview of Updated Evidence of Potential Health Risks,' *Korean Journal of Family Medicine*, vol. 41, no. 6, pp. 365-373, 2020, https://www.ncbi.nlm.nih.gov/pmc/articles/PMC7700832/

M Sisson, *The Primal Blueprint: Reprogram your genes for effortless weight loss, vibrant health and boundless energy*. Ebury Digital, 2012.

B Choi et al., 'Daily step goal of 10,000 steps: a literature review,' *Clinical Investigation Medicine*, vol. 30, no. 3, pp. 146-151, 2007, https://pubmed.ncbi.nlm.nih.gov/17716553/

C Tudor-Locke, 'Steps to Better Cardiovascular Health: How Many Steps Does It Take to Achieve Good Health and How Confident Are We in This Number?', *Curr Cardiovascular Risk Rep*, vol. 4, no. 4, pp. 271-276, 2010, https://www.ncbi.nlm.nih.gov/pmc/articles/PMC2894114/

T Morrison, *Chronic Fatigue Syndrome: A guide to recovery*. Palmer Higgs, 2013.

Chapter 10: Restorative Movement

M Caine, The Breakthrough Institute, https://thebreakthrough.org/people/mark-caine

J Clear, *Atomic Habits: An Easy & Proven Way to Build Good Habits & Break Bad Ones*. Cornerstone Digital, 2018.

J Berardi, *Precision Nutrition System*, 2009.

L Vartanian et al., 'Clutter, Chaos, and Overconsumption: The Role of Mind-Set in Stressful and Chaotic Food Environments,' *Environment and Behaviour*, 2016, https://papers.ssrn.com/sol3/papers.cfm?abstract_id=2711870

I Darien, 'People at risk of hoarding disorder may have serious complaints about sleep,' American Academy of Sleep Medicine, 2015, https://www.eurekalert.org/news-releases/612155

D Saxbe & R Repetti, 'No Place Like Home: Home Tours Correlate With Daily Patterns of Mood and Cortisol,' *Sage Journals*, vol. 36, no. 1, 2009, https://journals.sagepub.com/doi/abs/10.1177/0146167209352864

C Roster & J Ferrari, 'Does Work Stress Lead to Office Clutter, and How? Mediating Influences of Emotional Exhaustion and Indecision,' Sage Journals, vol. 52, no. 9, 2019, https://journals.sagepub.com/doi/abs/10.1177/0013916518823041?casa_token=yQLToPTHinAAAAAA:MgAqBDvc_MlH7UAWMZqtKLy1ZP7Rtr_SF0c_OnN20oPQuo89W5U8ucPHg6gjwShwy430Pj2tytLc

Chapter 11: Low Tox Home

'Scientists categorize Earth as a 'toxic planet',' *SciNews*, 2017, https://phys.org/news/2017-02-scientists-categorize-earth-toxic-planet.html

L Cohen & A Jefferies, 'Environmental exposures and cancer: using the precautionary principle,' E Cancer Medical Science, vol. 13, no. 91, 2019, https://www.ncbi.nlm.nih.gov/pmc/articles/PMC6546253/

S Yang et al, 'The Effects of Environmental Toxins on Allergic Inflammation,' Allergy Asthma Immunology Research, vol. 6, no. 6, pp. 478-484, 2014, https://www.ncbi.nlm.nih.gov/pmc/articles/PMC4214967/

H Lahouaoui et al., 'Depression and Anxiety Emerging From Heavy Metals: What Relationship?' *Research Gate*, 2019, https://www.researchgate.net/publication/330635466_Depression_and_Anxiety_Emerging_From_Heavy_Metals_What_Relationship

R Mason, 'Environmental Toxins and Weight Gain: The Link. An Interview with Paula Baillie-Hamilton MB, BS, Dphil,' Environmental, vol. 120, 2006, http://www.positivehealth.com/article/environmental/environmental-toxins-and-weight-gain-the-link-an-interview-with-paula-baillie-hamilton-mb-bs-dphil

E Erhirhie et al., 'Advances in acute toxicity testing: strengths, weaknesses and regulatory acceptance,' *Interdisciplinary Toxcology*, vol. 11, no. 1, pp. 5-12, 2018, https://www.ncbi.nlm.nih.gov/pmc/articles/PMC6117820/

P Darbe et al., 'Concentrations of parabens in human breast tumours,' *Journal of Applied Toxicology*, vol. 24, no. 1, pp. 5-13, 2004, https://centaur.reading.ac.uk/10465/

Think Dirty app, https://thinkdirtyapp.com/

B Statham & L Schneider, *The Chemical Maze: Your Guide to Food Additives and Cosmetic Ingredients*, 2012.

Environmental Working Group, www.ewg.org

T Miah & D Kamat, 'Current Understanding of the Health Effects of Electromagnetic Fields,' Pediatric Ann., vol. 46, no. 4, pp. 172e-174, 2017, https://pubmed.ncbi.nlm.nih.gov/28414399/

D Carpenter, 'Human disease resulting from exposure to electromagnetic fields,' *Rev Environmental Health*, vol. 28, no. 4, pp. 159-172, 2013, https://pubmed.ncbi.nlm.nih.gov/24280284/

G Chevalier et al., 'Earthing: Health Implications of Reconnecting the Human Body to the Earth's Surface Electrons,' J*ournal of Environmental Public Health*, 2012, https://www.ncbi.nlm.nih.gov/pmc/articles/PMC3265077/

K Goodwin, *Dear Digital, We Need To Talk: A Guilt-Free Guide To Taming Your Tech Habits and Thriving in a Distracted World*. Major Street Publishing, 2023.

V Valtonen, 'Clinical Diagnosis of the Dampness and Mold Hypersensitivity Syndrome: Review of the Literature and Suggested Diagnostic Criteria,' *Frontiers in Immunology*, vol. 8, no. 951, 2017, https://www.ncbi.nlm.nih.gov/pmc/articles/PMC5554125/

Chapter 12: Happy Home

M Reblin, 'Social and Emotional Support and its Implication for Health,' Curr. Opin. Psychiatry, vol. 21, vol. 2, pp. 201-205, 2009, https://www.ncbi.nlm.nih.gov/pmc/articles/PMC2729718/

J Frazer, *Leverage: How to change the people you love for all the right reasons and get the relationships you deserve*. Major Street Publishing, 2022.

'The Household, Income and Labour Dynamics in Australia (HILDA) Survey,' *Melbourne Institute Applied Economic and Social Research*, 2022, https://melbourneinstitute.unimelb.edu.au/hilda

S Karpman, *A Game Free Life: The definitive book on the Drama Triangle and Compassionate Triangle*. Drama Triangle Publications, 2014

Appendix

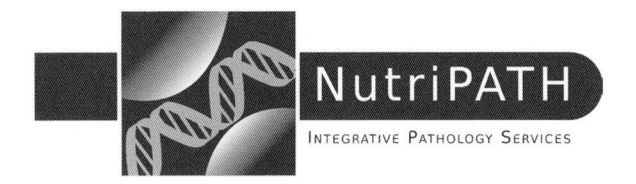

Lab Testing

My lab company of choice is Nutripath. Here's a list of all labs mentioned in the book:

- AdrenoCortex Stress Profile (1001)
- Organic Acids Metabolic Mapping (4041)
- Female Cycle (28 Day) Hormone Profile (1004)
- Complete Microbiome Mapping (2206)
- S.I.B.O. Breath Test (2025)
- Vaginal Microbiome Profile (2031)
- MTHFR Gene Mutation (5018)
- NutriStat (5005)
- Allergy Panels – IgE 15 Moulds Blood SST (3203)

Nutripath functional lab testing is available via accredited practitioners. Speak to your practitioner about ordering a test. If you're a practitioner, go to the Nutripath website for more information - www.nutripath.com.au

A big thank you to Nutripath for proudly sponsoring the publication of this book.

Acknowledgements

This book baby has been growing inside me for at least the last 10 years. But if I'm being really honest, the story started right back when I was a little girl. There have been many people who have been part of this ending body burnout story, and many people who have helped birth my book into being.

    First and foremost, massive gratitude to my hubby and business partner Chris Bellette. The principles, frameworks & advice in this book are as much yours as they are mine. Without you and your big vision and your natural ability to push the boundaries of "ordinary," this book and our Ending Body Burnout Method would not exist. Thank you for (often challenging!) conversations that have pushed me to think bigger and better, and for being my growth buddy and lover in life.

    To our two beautiful daughters, Poppy and Elsie. The birth of you both were the catalyst for my epic journey towards health and life. I have loved your input and your genuine interest in helping Mum with her book.

To all of our clients over the past 15 years since working in the health industry. You are the life of our Ending Body Burnout Method. Every one of you have helped us develop and tweak our method to become what it is today. Thank you for trusting us to be your guide, for being our beta-testers (in the early days!), and for leaning into the process of becoming your own self-healer and creating the body and the life of your dreams.

A very big thank you to our mentors and coaches who have played a pivotal role in the creation of this book - Dr Daniel Kalish, Dr Nirala Jacobi, Dr Jason Hawrelak, Jaemin Frazer, Kylie Ryan, Glen Carlson and the team at Dent Global. We truly stand on the shoulders of giants!

Also much gratitude to my book sponsors - Nutripath and Helen from Primal Alternative. You saw the potential of this book, and so generously backed me. And to my beta-readers who gave up their time when the book was only in its messy second draft - Erica Mansfield, Alanna Kirkwood, Sally Milbourne, Elizabeth Diacos, Katie Tangney and Emily Johnson. Thank you for both the kind encouragement and your brutal feedback (which only made this book better). Also to my book endorsers - Lisa Corduff, Dr Kristy Goodwin, Lorraine Murphy and Jeannie Savage. You are all inspiring female entrepreneurs, authors and speakers in your own right!

To my publishing team from Book Reality, especially Ian Hooper and Krysta Micallef, who worked meticulously to bring my scribbles into a professional book. And also to the Book Builder team from Rethink Press. Your process squashed out any writer's block, allowing me to get my first draft written in an unbelievable 6-weeks.

And finally, a massive thanks to you! Thank you for investing time from your "busy" life to read my words. I wrote this book for you, because I believe YOU CAN HEAL. In a world of Dr Google and lots of noise and confusion, I want you to know that there are only so many ways the body falls apart. Body burnout isn't a mystery. This book unlocks the structure of how and why your body burns out, and what to do to restore it. I'm cheering you on all the way!

Sponsor Appreciation

Last but certainly not least, I'd also love to give a big thanks to Nutripath, functional lab testing, Primal Alternative, wholefood grain-free products, and Happy Biome, natural skincare & cleaning products, for sponsoring the publication of this book. Check these awesome companies out!

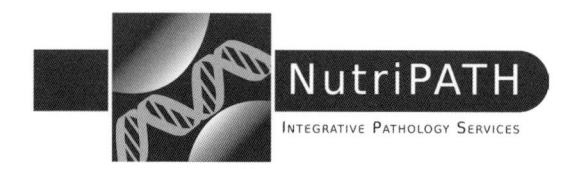

Nutripath
www.nutripath.com.au

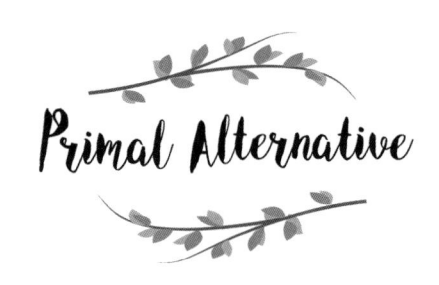

Primal Alternative
www.primalalternative.com

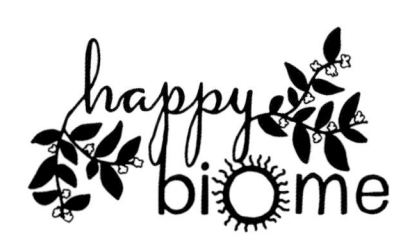

Happy Biome
www.happybiome.com.au

The Author

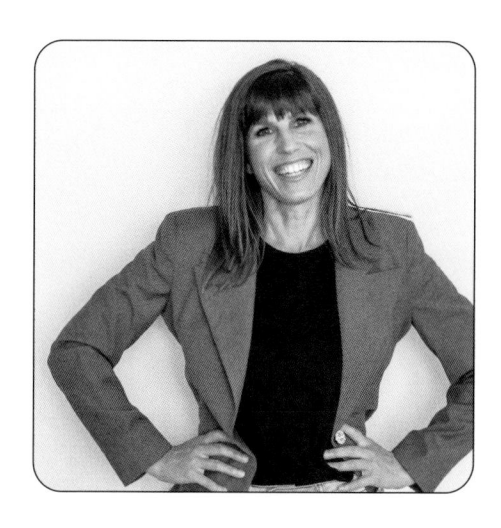

Filipa Bellette is co-founder of multi award-winning health practice Chris & Filly Functional Medicine. She is an accredited Clinical Nutritionist, Functional Medicine Practitioner, Coach & Trauma Therapist. She is also a PhD Scholar, award-winning writer & regularly featured in the media, such as Forbes, Body+Soul and nine.com.au

Together with her husband Chris Bellette (contributing author to this book), Filipa has worked with over 2,000+ burned-out women and men in the past combined 25+ years. Their practice is best known for ending body burnout (for good!) in "busy" people with energy, mood & gut issues. They were recently awarded as the Tasmanian State Winner & National Finalist for the Telstra Best of Business Awards 2022, as well as Winner for the Australian Women's Small Business Champion Awards 2022.

Filipa's own passion for helping "busy" people have more energy, productivity and connection, came from her own personal experience of body burnout, after juggling the demands of business, family, and her failing health.

Connect with Filipa online here:
Website   www.chrisandfilly.fm
Facebook   www.facebook.com/chrisandfilly
Instagram   @chrisandfilly_fm

And for book resources mentioned in the book, go here: www.chrisandfilly.fm/book

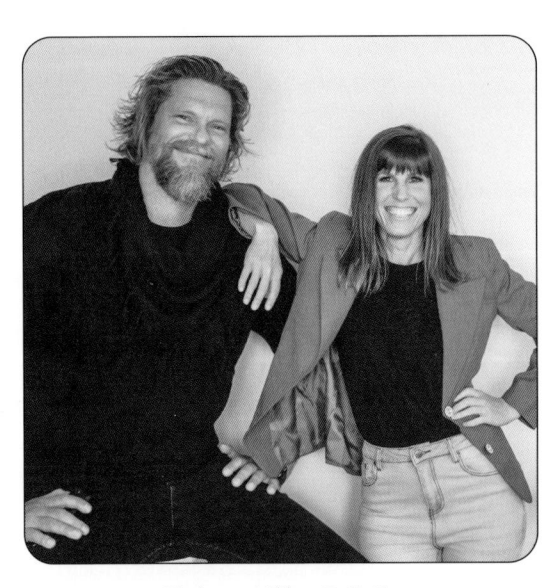

Chris and Filipa Bellette

ARE YOU PASSIONATE ABOUT HEALTHY EATING AND BAKING?
DO YOU DREAM OF BEING YOUR OWN BOSS AND WORKING FROM HOME?

Then why not explore becoming a Primalista with Primal Alternative!

Our grain-free, gluten-free food products are loved by health enthusiasts all over Australia, and with our Primalista Licence, you can join our mission to make healthy home-made food easy and accessible for people in your community.

As a Primalista, you'll have the freedom to work around your family and follow your joy while creating a lifestyle full of the things you love.

You can work from your own kitchen and build a business that fits your unique vision and goals. Plus, you'll be part of a larger wellness community that includes like-minded Primalistas and collaboration with Chris & Filly, Jo Whitton from Quirky Cooking, and Alexx Stuart from Low Tox Life.

But being a Primalista isn't just about the freedom to work from home and follow your passion - it's also about the satisfaction of creating delicious, healthy treats that your customers will love. Our food products are all grain-free, making them naturally gluten-free, and we also offer plant-based, nut-free, GAPS-friendly, and low-carb options to cater to different dietary needs. You'll be proud to offer a range of options that cater to a variety of tastes and dietary requirements.

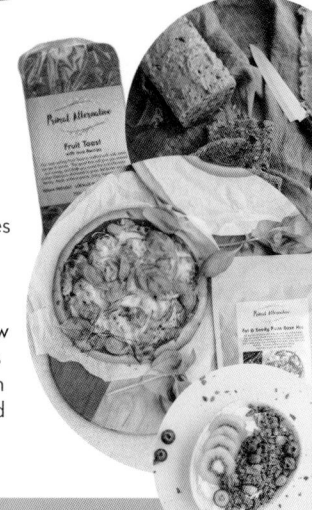

SCAN THE QR CODE

Or visit https://training.primalalternative.com/info-pack to download our free info pack, including a Grain-Free Herb Bread recipe to try at home.

With the Primalista Licence, you'll receive comprehensive training, ongoing support and all the tools you need to start and grow your business. You'll be your own boss, follow your passion and create a lifestyle that works for you and your family.

Join the Primalista movement today and discover how easy it is to make grain-free a part of your life while building a successful business doing what you love!

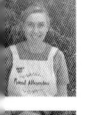

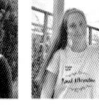

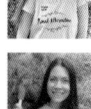

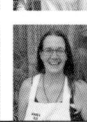

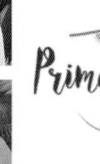

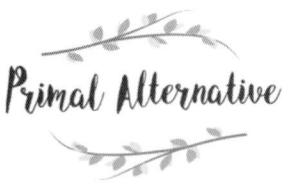

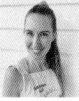

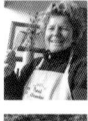

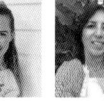

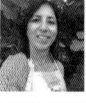

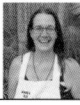

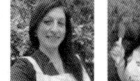

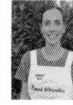

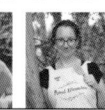

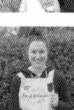

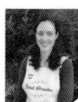

Primal Alternative